The Obvious Diet

Ed Victor

The Obvious Diet

Ed Victor

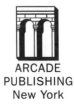

ARCADE
PUBLISHING
New York

FIRST NORTH AMERICAN EDITION 2002

First published in 2001, in the U.K. by Vermilion, an imprint of Ebury Press, Random House U.K. Ltd.

Library of Congress Cataloging-in-Publication Data

    Victor, Ed.
      The obvious diet / Ed Victor. —1st North American ed.
        p. cm.
      Includes bibliographical references and index.
      ISBN 1-55970-651-1
        1. Reducing diets. I. Title.
    RM222.2 .V495 2002
    613.2'5—dc21   2002071730

Published in the United States by Arcade Publishing, Inc., New York

Distributed by AOL Time Warner Book Group

Visit our Web site at www.arcadepub.com

10 9 8 7 6 5 4 3 2 1

EB

PRINTED IN THE UNITED STATES OF AMERICA

To Carol

Contents

Foreword

Ed Victor may have written *The Obvious Diet*, but
– thank God – he isn't the obvious dieter. I have
heard him on the subject of chicken skin, blister-
ing gold and crisp, oozing juices. I have eaten with
him in Chinatown and seen the waiter's look of
awe and respect turn, after two tablefuls of food,
to panicked disbelief. His claim to be "one of the
greediest eaters I know" is no idle one – for
which, maximum respect – and consequently
when he adds "if I can do it, anyone can" I am
prepared to believe him. Who, anyway, would trust
a man who found the renouncing of the flesh
easy?

True, I don't declare myself to be altogether ready to follow
him on the path to dietary virtue, but I am convinced –
convinced enough to let him do it on my behalf. Just as many

people read cookbooks in order to consume food without the calorie intake, I am a believer in the vicarious diet. But the point of Ed is not that he is an evangelist, but an enthusiast. He doesn't preach; he has just found a way of being as exuberant about resistance as he normally is about indulgence.

Anyway, why should someone lose weight without suffering? That small, sweet mean-spirited voice inside of me likes it that he hasn't given up without a struggle. I exult in his mournful comparison of the Sacred Heart Memorial Hospital 7 Day Fat Burning Diet's Cabbage Soup (of Cabbage Soup Diet fame) to his mother's borscht, "full of the fatty juices of the flanken beef she used for the stock and … served with a large dollop of sour cream." I wallow in his confession that giving up cheese, on the advice of the nutritional guru Dr. Ali, is "a blow from which I am still trying to recover." I smile when I read that giving up bacon and sausages at breakfast was "one of my greatest personal sacrifices." This, surely, is how it should be.

A diet that works doesn't have to make sense to everyone, but it has to make sense to the person who follows it.

I don't say this entirely meanly. The duty of a diet book may well be to inspire, but those of us who resist inspiration need to be rewarded too. I remember once being entirely heartened by an interview with Cindy Crawford in which she outlined her exercise routine and itemized her food intake. It helps to know that in order to look like Cindy Crawford you need to exercise four times a week and live on grilled skinned chicken portions and steamed vegetables. Because if that's what it takes, no thank you: it's too high a price. The chapter in *The Obvious Diet* called How They Do It: The Secrets of Famous People offers more comfort in this vein. A life spent going to restaurants and ordering Dover sole is no life at all, as Anne Robinson dryly notes. That's not just why I like this chapter, though.

This chapter underlines the strength of Ed's dietary approach. A diet that works doesn't have to make sense to everyone, but it has to make sense to the person who follows it.

Most diet books infantilize the reader; they induce nervous dependence rather than confidence. Anyone who knows Ed knows too that inducing confidence is, above all, his strength. And this book shares the giddy virtues of its author: it's lively, insistently pleasure-seeking, and absurdly encouraging.

Nigella Lawson

Introduction

When my old friend and sometime literary agent Ed Victor told me that he was writing a book about the diet plan he devised for himself, I was delighted for more than one reason. Ed, like me, grew up in New York in the forties. He was raised in the Bronx, and his Russian-Jewish mother was a world-class cook. He knows good food. We have shared many fine meals together.

But Ed ventured far from home as a young man. He won a scholarship to Cambridge, got his master's degree in literature, and forged a distinguished career in publishing. After a brief return to New York in the early seventies, where he met his wife, the lovely lawyer Carol, he returned to Britain for good. He founded the Ed Victor Literary Agency in 1976, and has since flourished as Britain's most formidable, and most famous, literary agent. His clients include Nigella Lawson, England's reigning domestic goddess; Anne Robinson, Jack Higgins, Erica Jong, Frederick Forsyth, Erich Segal, and

Andrew Lloyd Webber; he also oversees the estates of such writers as Raymond Chandler, Irving Wallace, and Iris Murdoch.

Ed is a renowned bon vivant and gourmand in his adopted hometown of London. Ed had always been frank about his love of eating, and let's face it, literary agents are famous for their long lunches, replete with wine and dessert. His life is a relentless social whirl of cocktail parties, book launches, and business lunches, most often at the world's finest restaurants. A couple of years ago I ran into Ed, as I periodically do. I was amazed at his noticeable weight loss. He proudly informed me that he had shed more

If he could do it, living the lifestyle he did, he assured me anyone could.

than forty pounds on a plan of his own making. This got my attention. If he could do it, living the lifestyle he did, he assured me anyone could.

His premise grabbed me immediately. Using your common sense, most of us know exactly what it would take to lose a significant amount of weight in a short time. We could do it easily if we had sufficient desire. Anyone over a certain age – say twenty-five – knows exactly what makes them fat and what kind of diet and exercise program keeps them slim. We all know our own bodies intimately; each person is his own best expert. Ed succeeded in losing weight by designing his own diet and policing it himself, not following the dictates of whatever new plan was fashionable. People follow the rules they make themselves. This philosophy is the cornerstone to The Obvious Diet.

I was not the only one to take notice that his plan was effective. His various friends and clients shared personal recipes, diet tips, and strategies learned along the way, as you will see in Chapter Eight. And soon enough the agent decided to become an author. The shoe was on the other foot for Ed this time. Although he is notorious as a fearless and tough negotiator, he was now a vulnerable and insecure author.

I think that besides producing a great book, this has been a valuable learning experience for this master of the game.

I know you'll enjoy all the recipes and advice in this great book (look out for my special tuna salad!). Forget all the rules you've heard about what to eat and get inspired for a whole new you: at last, The Obvious Diet has arrived.

Larry King

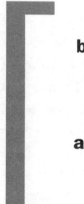

The Obvious Diet is based on my firm belief that it is far easier to ignore an outside authority than rules you create yourself.

Ed Victor

CHAPTER ONE

Why The Obvious Diet Works

Like most people I know, my weight has always been a problem that needs constant attention. The publishing world in which I swim lives as much by its stomach as it does by its brains. Publishing lunches are famous, and so are the launch parties with their endless champagne and canapés. And although we have proclaimed "the death of the dinner party," evenings dining out in restaurants or eating store-bought prepared meals are now the norm rather than the exception and contribute inevitably to an ever-expanding waistline.

I didn't know whether to laugh or cry when a *Daily Express* reporter caught up with me at my Long Island summer home a couple of years ago to tell me my wife, Carol, and I were number two on the *Tatler* list of "the most invited people in London." My profession as literary agent to many famous authors and celebrities inevitably leads me to many high-powered social functions — not to mention business breakfasts and working lunches at some of the finest res-taurants and hotels in London, New York, and Los Angeles.

But was I *really* that much of a party animal? The answer was clearly "yes" – since only Elton John was ahead of me on the list! – and I'm afraid my growing paunch was more than ample testimony to the truth about the high life I was leading.

What did I do? Like everybody else, I went on diets. Sometimes it would be the Hay Diet (food combining), sometimes the Atkins Diet (high protein, low carbohydrate). Then there are the various "samizdat" diets, crumpled Xeroxed sheets passed from hand to hand with the details of the Mayo Clinic Diet or the Sacred Heart Memorial Hospital 7 Day Fat Burning Diet (aka the Cabbage Soup Diet). The latest food fetishes come in like clockwork. Every year, more and more diets are published, either as books or in the January editions of Sunday supplements. And the one thing they all have in common is this: people stop observing them almost as soon as they start. Even if dieters do manage to follow these regimens to their conclusions, the weight lost simply flies back on at the end, because "normal" eating and drinking patterns are reestablished all too quickly.

So, diets don't work. Why? Because, like buses, they are "hop-on, hop-off" experiences.

Diets don't work. Why? Because, like buses, they are "hop-on, hop-off" experiences.

When I was in Los Angeles recently, I was struck by the frequency of diet ads on the television and radio. I heard about diets that promised women they would "lose one dress size over the weekend," or even diets that would guarantee you "lose weight while you sleep!" The fundamental problem with all these "lose-weight-quick" schemes is that they deal more or less exclusively in abstention: avoid this food and that drink for a few days/weeks and all will be well. Not true. In 99.9 percent of cases, all these diets achieve is the familiar spiral of putting on weight and then going back on diets. They focus on short-term prohibitions – what you cannot eat – instead of long-term goals: what you can eat to stay slim, fit, and healthy.

About five years ago, I went on a diet of my own devising (and therefore my own policing!) during the course of which I lost a very noticeable amount of weight. One day, when a publisher friend remarked on my new slim-line look, he asked me what diet I was on. Without thinking, I replied: "The Obvious Diet." "What's that?" he asked. I said that everybody over a certain age (let's say about thirty, though many younger people have plenty of yo-yo dieting experience) knows very well what foods make them fat and what kind of eating regime helps keeps them slim. It's obvious! Whereupon he offered me a publishing contract, which I politely refused, thinking that I – much more a sinner than a saint when it comes to food – was surely the wrong person to preach publicly about restraint in eating. And sure enough, after about a year of being good and more or less religiously following the eating parameters I had so successfully established for myself, I fell off the wagon – right back into the kind of greedy, thoughtless eating that gave rise to my old weight problems.

Last autumn, during the course of the illness and death of a close family member, my eating actually reached crisis point. I realized that not only was I making my normal, highly sybaritic professional and social rounds, but also indulging in what is called "comfort eating." At the height (or should I say depth) of my comfort eating phase, I put away more food than I could possibly have needed: "Hmm, that was a good cheeseburger, I think I'll have another, thank you very much. And, oh, by the way, could you please bring me some more fries while you're at it?" I couldn't believe how much food I was gulping down, hating myself for doing it while, at the same time, feeling compelled to just carry on eating. It was, like smoking too many cigarettes or drinking too much alcohol, an addiction run wild. The weight flew on and on, until I decided to return to "The Obvious Diet," which had served me so well a few years earlier. This time around, however, my Obvious Diet has become a plan for life. The second time a publisher offered me a contract for the diet, I had run out of reasons to refuse. This book is the result of that decision.

You know what makes you fat, just as you know how to lose weight.

The Obvious Diet is based on my firm belief that it is far easier to ignore an outside authority than rules you create yourself and the tenets of your own conscience. As I have said, you know what makes you fat, just as you know how to lose weight.

You know when you are eating for comfort, or when you are succumbing to a craving that has nothing to do with your dietary needs. Nobody knows more about yourself than you do: you are the world's No. 1 expert. You're also the one who knows how much you really want to lose weight, and you have the experience of all the ways you have tried over the years to solve your weight problems once and for all. You are unquestionably your own prime motivator. Were I to say to any male friend that he could costar in a movie with Julia Roberts or Michelle Pfeiffer on condition that he lost twenty pounds in four weeks, he would know exactly what to do, what to eat and what not to eat, in order to shed that weight, without consulting a single diet book or article (for women, cast Tom Cruise or Brad Pitt as the hypothetical leading man!). Our system is hardwired with this knowledge; it is just a question of accessing it, and this book will show you exactly how to do that.

There are many roads you can take to arrive at your ideal diet. Once you start thinking about it, it's obvious – we are all different, we all have our own needs. There is no "one-size-fits-all" diet solution. For example, I know that carbohydrates put weight on me, so therefore I need to avoid bread and pasta. I also know that my lifelong predilection for animal fat (sausage, bacon, and fatty meats in general) adds weight.

The Obvious Diet really works because it is designed to work just for you! I am one of the greediest eaters I know, so if I can do it, anybody can. All it really takes is the setting of a goal that is already in your own mind and within your own capabilities, drawing upon your own experience – not somebody else's. The rest is obvious!

In Chapter Two, Before Getting Started, I will tell you exactly how to go about finding a nutritionist and obtaining the information you need in order to initiate your own Obvious Diet, specially tailored to your own nutritional needs. When I went to a nutritionist, I was informed (for the first time in my life!) that I was averse to wheat, yeast, and gluten, so pasta and bread (with its animal-fat partner, butter) had to go out of my life. A good friend, the American actress Gayle Hunnicutt, was suffering for years from chronic fatigue, especially after eating. Endless doctors offered her no cure, until finally she went to see a nutritionist, who told her to cut wheat, yeast, sugar, and vinegar out of her diet. Like flicking a switch, Gayle's health and energy returned overnight as a result of these simple dietary steps. In my case, eating bread or pasta didn't provoke a violent reaction; far from it. But I had been suffering a feeling of great heaviness after eating a meal containing wheat or gluten. Life has become much more pleasant now that those things have been cut out. Very often a little nutritional self-knowledge can have a hugely beneficial effect on your sense of physical well-being.

One of the advantages of The Obvious Diet is that you can mix and match elements from any other diet regime. For example, I use the Cabbage Soup recipe from the Sacred Heart Memorial Hospital 7 Day Fat Burning Diet for my "Cleansing Day" – about which more later. Diet veterans know which diets are hideous and intolerable torture; conversely, anybody who has dieted has personal experience of what principles have worked in the past at not too much cost in terms of physical and mental well-being. The Obvious Diet provides you with a list of the best-known diets on the market, each with their salient points succinctly outlined.

> **Very often a little nutritional self-knowledge can have a hugely beneficial effect on your sense of physical well-being.**

The idea is for you to choose – and use – what you like about each eating plan, adapt and incorporate information from your nutritional detective work, and then raid your store of cookbooks and recipes to find delicious meals that fit the diet you have devised for yourself.

No scales, please! An important precept of The Obvious Diet for me is the banishing of all scales from the procedure. It is simply too disheartening to watch the numbers nudge down ever so slowly on a dial as the weeks go by. For me, the greatest reinforcement factor is in having your partner recognize, through a hug, how much less of you there seems to be. Not having to suck your gut in when a photograph is about to be taken is a great pleasure! And, day after day, people I haven't seen for a while comment on how slim I look. Believe me, these are far better rewards than watching a dial move a couple of notches downwards. (Although the no-scales rule is one I strongly recommend, if scale-gazing is an imperative part of how you monitor your eating habits, then there's no reason not to peek once in a while.)

There is another, immensely satisfying, tangible reward: the vast pleasure you can take in being able to easily button clothes that had been previously impossible to wear. Last New Year's Eve, unable to wear the suit I had laid out for the fashionable New York party I was attending, I made plans to go to my tailors, Anderson & Sheppard, in defeat to have the trousers let out. Now I have scheduled a visit to Savile Row in order to have them taken in!

Incidentally, at that New Year's Eve party, one of the guests was Mike Wallace, the 80+-year-old star of *60 Minutes*, looking twenty years younger and wonderfully slim and fit. My wife whispered in the ear of his wife: "What's his secret?" The answer was to the point: "He eats very, very little and exercises every day."

Exercise is another important factor in The Obvious Diet. This means getting into a program of exercise to complement your eating program and establishing a routine – *your* routine – for matching your dietary efforts with a minimum regimen of exercise. It can be a mixture of anything: a round of golf, a couple of sets of tennis, a brisk walk in the park, yoga, or whatever physical activity you enjoy and can do – *but you must do it at least three times each week*. My personal exercise regime is a one-hour mixture of stretching, aerobics, and weight training every Monday, Wednesday, and Friday before breakfast.

Exercise helps in so many ways: expending energy makes you feel better, it helps you tone up, and it provides you with a concrete measure of how much fitter you are becoming – far more reaffirming than those banished scales; it also helps keep your weight in check and makes you feel better about yourself. But, as with everything in The Obvious Diet, your exercise program can be exactly what you want it to be, tailored to fit in with your life, as long as you put in the minimum requirement of three times a week.

The Obvious Diet will help you listen to your body.

A word of warning is due here. People who tend to lead sedentary lives and are not used to taking exercise are always advised to seek advice from their physician or a trainer before beginning an exercise program, as sudden furious physical activity after a long period of inactivity is an almost sure-fire path to injury.

The Obvious Diet will show you how to establish your own individual eating plan and inspire you to keep to it. It will provide many sample recipes drawn from the recipes I use for my own Obvious Dieting. You are welcome to borrow them, but you may well be better off finding your own! There will also be advice about how not to cheat on yourself – as well as advice on when, how, and how often to cheat! One of the best things about The Obvious Diet, in my view, is that absolutely no foods are permanently banned. I will show you how to get ready to launch yourself into Obvious Dieting, how to deal with the "Cleansing Day" each week, and how to keep the weight off over the long run. My hope is to help you break free of the start-stop tyranny of ordinary diet regimens.

The Obvious Diet will help you listen to your body, search your soul, do some basic research to gather together the nutritional information you need, and then mix these ingredients into a coherent and systematic form – your own recipe for eating healthily, feeling good about your eating, and losing weight in the most long-term and effective way possible: YOUR OWN WAY!

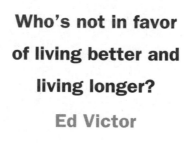

[
Who's not in favor
of living better and
living longer?
Ed Victor
]

CHAPTER TWO

Before Getting Started

When I started writing this book, this was the part
that filled me with the greatest trepidation. Like
you, I am a consumer – not a provider – of scientific information. In short, an absolute layman in
these matters. But with all the bad habits we may
have picked up, and all the potentially dubious
advice that, over the years, we may have garnered
from faddish diets, I feel it is important to present
here the results of my research into what constitutes a healthy, balanced, life-sustaining
nutritional diet. For instance, the surprising fact
that 60 percent of the human body by weight is
water, around 20 percent is fat, and just 20
percent is a combination of all the things we hear
about from nutritionists: protein, carbohydrates,
vitamins, and minerals. If this chapter is full of
things that you already know, all well and good –
much of what follows falls into the category of

common sense – you can skip to Chapter Three, Getting Started. I would, however, advise at least a cursory glance through the information I have put together – think of it as the initial blueprint for the edifice you are about to build.

First, though, some questions. How many times have you heard lectures about eating guidelines for the promotion of good health and weight management offered by nutritionists and dietitians? Or read an article in the newspaper about some new scientific research into eating habits? This is the moment to recap that knowledge. Before we get down to the business of bringing together the various elements that will make up your own personal Obvious Diet, get yourself a pad of paper – you're going to be using that pad a lot, I warn you right now – and write down the healthy eating principles you already know, things you have been taught, and ideas you may have overheard on television or read about in books – especially those that you feel apply particularly to you. This is a moment to go back to first principles, to build your Obvious Diet from the ground up in order to make it as solid as possible. On the topic of first principles, think about this: the Ancient Greek word from which we get the word diet, *diaita*, means simply "way of life."

Official Nutritional Guidelines

The first port of call in my journey of research was the land of officialdom. Obviously enough, as an American living permanently in England, I checked with health departments in both of my countries. It is fascinating to see how very close the two sets of guidelines are.

These guidelines have been issued as a kind of simplified roadmap for people who want to lead a healthy life. They recognize the pitfalls of living in our fast-paced, fast-food-oriented 21st-century world, and offer bare-bones advice for eating in such a way as to get at least the minimum nutrition an average adult requires to feel and stay healthy. Note the use of the word "average": this advice – in fact all general dietary advice – should be leavened with the unique requirements of the individual, which means *you*. This is why it is always a good idea to seek professional medical counsel when it comes to dietary measures. If you decide to start a new diet – this one or any other! – you should definitely talk to your GP about your plans. You need to make sure that your diet fits in with any special requirements you may have because of medical conditions or medicines you may be taking. You should also ask your physician about seeing a nutritionist or dietitian, about which more later.

British Health Education Authority's Healthy Living Unit Recommendations:

- Enjoy your food.

- Eat a variety of foods.

- Eat plenty of foods rich in starch and fiber.

- Don't eat too much fat.

- Don't eat sugary foods too often.

- Eat foods that provide enough vitamins and minerals.

- If you drink alcohol, drink sensibly.

- Eat the right amount to be a healthy weight.

U.S. Department of Agriculture and U.S. Department of Health and Human Services Dietary Guidelines for Americans:

- Eat a variety of foods.

- Balance the food you eat with physical activity to maintain or improve your weight.

- Choose a diet with plenty of grain products, vegetables, and fruits.

- Choose a diet low in fat, saturated fat, and cholesterol.

- Choose a diet moderate in sugars.

- Choose a diet moderate in salt and sodium.

- If you drink alcoholic beverages, do so in moderation.

The U.S. guidelines also include a sample breakdown of the five different food groups we should all eat within the span of a day. This is where it all starts to get technical, so if figures make you swoon, then turn the page and carry on from there:

Food Group	Recommended Servings per Day
Grains (bread, cereal, pasta, and rice)	6–11
Vegetables (whole vegetables and vegetable juices)	3–5
Fruits (whole fruits and fruit juices)	2–4
Milk products (milk, yogurt, and cheese)	2–3
Proteins (meat, poultry, fish, dry beans, eggs, and nuts)	2 3

To understand this obviously requires a chart of what constitutes a "serving portion," which you will find on the overleaf.

How much you actually need to consume to function well depends on the kind of life you lead. A man who spends his day doing heavy, physical work needs upwards of 3,000 calories a day, in other words the upper number of recommended servings; this is more or less twice the nutritional requirement of an average woman who leads a sedentary life. Incidentally, I was surprised to learn that a calorie is actually a measurement of the heat generated by the body from the food it has ingested, to use as energy. For your information, one gram of protein contains 4 calories, one gram of fat has 9 calories, one gram of carbohydrates is worth 4 calories. Of

Food Group	Serving Size
Bread	1 slice
Cereal	1 ounce ready-to-eat or 1 cup cooked cereal
Pasta and rice	4 ounces cooked pasta or rice
Vegetables	8 ounces raw leafy vegetables or 4 ounces chopped raw or cooked vegetables or 4 tablespoons vegetable juice
Fruits	1 piece of fresh fruit or 1/2 cup cooked or canned fruit or 1/2 cup fruit juice
Dairy products	1 cup milk or 1 cup yogurt or 1 ounce cheese
Meat	2 or 3 ounces lean cooked weight
Poultry	2 or 3 ounces lean cooked weight
Fish	2 or 3 ounces lean cooked weight
Dry beans	1/2 cup cooked
Eggs	1
Nuts	3 tablespoons
Fats, oils, and sweets	keep to a minimum

these, fat and meat maintain a feeling of fullness for longest, because they take longest to digest. This also means that they stave off hunger for longer. Alcohol weighs in at 7 calories per gram. Alcohol, like sugar, is known to nutritionists as an "empty-calorie" food, which means that apart from the calories they provide for conversion to energy, they bring no additional nutrients to help the body thrive.

What all this preamble boils down to, in the view of the U.S. authorities, is that we should be obtaining up to 60 percent of our daily calorie intake from carbohydrates (grains, legumes, bread, pasta, root vegetables, etc.), no more than 30 percent from fat, and less than 10 percent from protein (dairy products, meat, fish, etc.).

If you have trouble dealing with these figures, an alternative way to take in the general guidelines is through the Food Pyramid shown on the next page, another product of the U.S. Department of Agriculture/U.S. Department of Health and Human Services. This is a visual interpretation of the same nutritional guidelines as above.

Obviously, the larger blocks in the pyramid represent larger quantities. Once again, the suggested servings range from about 1,600 calories per day to over 3,000.

All dietary advice should be leavened with the unique requirements of the individual – you.

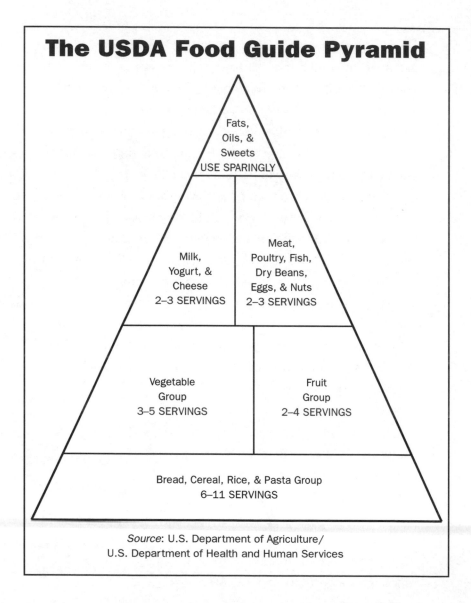

The USDA Food Guide Pyramid

Fats,
Oils, &
Sweets
USE SPARINGLY

Milk,
Yogurt, &
Cheese
2–3 SERVINGS

Meat,
Poultry, Fish,
Dry Beans,
Eggs, & Nuts
2–3 SERVINGS

Vegetable
Group
3–5 SERVINGS

Fruit
Group
2–4 SERVINGS

Bread, Cereal, Rice, & Pasta Group
6–11 SERVINGS

Source: U.S. Department of Agriculture/
U.S. Department of Health and Human Services

The World Health Organization has also published its own Food Pyramid, based upon the Mediterranean Diet (see following page). As you would expect, there is quite a contrast between the U.S. pyramid and the Mediterranean one. The main difference is that, rather than the red meat and dairy-heavy U.S. diet, the Mediterranean Food Pyramid gives greater prominence to grains and cereals, olive oil in substitution for butter (a standard practice in my own Obvious Diet, as you will see), relatively low consumption of dairy products, and a preference for fish and white meat. Proponents of this kind of diet point to studies that show the residents of Italy, Greece, and Spain have longer life expectancies than Americans, not to mention a lower incidence of heart disease and certain cancers of the digestive tract. Who's not in favor of living better and living longer?

One interesting way to work out which foods you should be eating to stay healthy is to build your own Food Pyramid: copy the outline and then fill in actual foods you eat (including some of your favorite foods) for the suggested groups. All very sensible, all very "obvious," very expert and very useful.

But what counts most here is what you in your bones know to be the right advice for you. For example, it is worth

What counts most here is what you in your bones know to be the right advice for you.

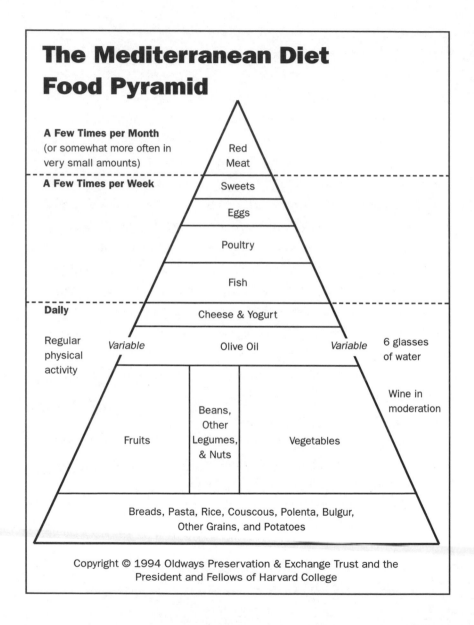

The Mediterranean Diet Food Pyramid

A Few Times per Month
(or somewhat more often in
very small amounts)

Red Meat

A Few Times per Week

Sweets

Eggs

Poultry

Fish

Daily

Cheese & Yogurt

Regular physical activity

Variable   Olive Oil   *Variable*

6 glasses of water

Wine in moderation

Fruits

Beans, Other Legumes, & Nuts

Vegetables

Breads, Pasta, Rice, Couscous, Polenta, Bulgur, Other Grains, and Potatoes remembering that everyone has a different body shape. As long as your weight is within the range advised by the medical community for your height and age, you are not overweight – even if you might feel that, from an aesthetic point of view, you are not slim enough.

Advice from Nutritional Scientists

Dietitians on both sides of the Atlantic unanimously advise eating as much fresh fruit and vegetables as possible, and generally steering clear of processed foods. Five portions of fresh fruit and vegetables per day, runs the mantra, and then your body will get its full requirement of vitamins and minerals – without having to resort to supplements.

One key precept above all others – especially if you are set to revamp the types and combinations of foods you consume – is that what you buy is naturally tasty. Even with the best will in the world, if the fruit and vegetables (not to mention the meat and fish) you bring home from the shops are tasteless and watery, you are going to find it very hard to stick to your new regime. My advice is to buy your fresh produce from a specialist outlet, such as a health food

Five portions of fresh fruit and vegetables per day – that's the mantra.

store, or one of the many companies that delivers a box of seasonal vegetables every week. Supermarkets are improving all the time, but I still find that in many cases their alluring displays are more about looks than substance.

Taste is also the best yardstick for gauging how much or how little meddling has been involved in the growing of your vegetables and fruit: if it has seen the sun and not been forced or placed in cold storage for a lengthy period, that apple is likely to burst with apple flavor. It's not for nothing that both the U.S. and U.K. health authorities preach avoidance of high sugar- and sodium- and fat-content foods, which is, it seems to me, a euphemistic way of saying prepackaged processed items. What's really wrong with processed foods – those generally brightly colored handy, convenient little packages of sustenance that are so simple to heat in a microwave? Well, lots of things, a lot of the time: too much salt, too much sugar, unidentifiable ingredients, preservatives, and food that has been stripped of all its nutritional goodness. Little wonder, then, that there have been such strong concerns about industrial farming methods and greater public awareness of organic produce.

This is why it's important to read the labels on the food you buy. There's little point in making a Herculean effort to eat right only to fill up on heaps of sugar and fats concealed in an outwardly inoffensive little snack bar. These nutritional baddies can lurk in unexpected places: animal fats feature in industrial quantities in many pre-prepared convenience foods, and salt is often present in abundance in foods that are advertised as low-fat. Remember, ingredients are always listed in order, the largest amounts first, so if fats, sugars, and salt are the opening things you see on a list of ingredients, the smart thing to do is to put whatever you are holding back on the shelf and look for a healthier alternative.

As seen on page 23, one of the key general rules suggested by nutritional scientists is that the lion's share (60 percent) of our calorie intake should come from carbohydrates. There are two types of carbohydrates: sugars (simple carbohydrates) and starches (complex carbohydrates), each of which can be found in two forms, natural or refined. It is the complex carbohydrates that are the good guys. These natural starches are found in whole grain breakfast cereals, whole-grain flour and bread, brown rice, potatoes, oats, lentils, bananas, and root vegetables. The theory behind this – bear with me if you know this already – is that the starches release their sugars into the bloodstream slowly, and therefore keep the body's energy levels in equilibrium (translation: no sudden peaks of energy and troughs of exhaustion). These plant-based foods are also a great delivery system for vitamins and minerals, and are naturally very low in fat.

On the other hand, refined sugars (in cakes, cookies, soft drinks, etc.) and refined starches (in white flour, sugary processed breakfast cereals, white rice, etc.) are the ones we are advised to avoid. They are absorbed by the body more quickly, so energy levels rise dramatically in the short term. However, the downside (there had to be one) is that the pancreas then produces more insulin in a bid to break down the sugar, which in turn leads to an equally dramatic slump in energy. All obvious stuff, but one of the real advantages of The Obvious Diet is that it should improve your overall health by getting you out of the habit of reaching for quick-fix refined-carb snacks – see how your energy levels soar as a result.

Most nutritionists – but not most diets I have tried – agree that tea and coffee are highly destabilizing to digestive functions. Not only are they stimulants, they cause blood sugar levels to fluctuate and, of course, they are addictive. Far better to drink a glass of water when you feel thirsty than automatically flick the switch on the kettle – and the best way to start the day, according to many life-diet practitioners, is with a cup of hot water and lemon to awaken the system gently.

Wolfing something down prevents you from savoring the flavors that made you start eating in the first place.

Other "obvious" nutritional guidelines abound. Those who find it hard to shed excess weight could do worse than follow the advice that so many mothers give their hungry children as they wolf down their evening meal: "eat slowly!" Careful chewing not only aids the whole process of digestion; it also allows the body to start sending signals that the appetite has been satisfied. Wolfing something down prevents you from savoring the flavors that made you start eating in the first place, and prevents the body from naturally recognizing that its hunger has been satisfied.

Ideal eating times vary from person to person – no Nobel Prize necessary to know that! – but the majority of scientific literature on the topic regards it as beneficial to consume a larger proportion of our daily food intake earlier in the day, that is to say a substantial breakfast and lunch as the biggest meal of the day, the theory being that these

Ideal eating times vary from person to person.

calories are processed and burned up when we need them most. Eating a big, heavy dinner may fit in better with our social or family arrangements, but it is also a perfect way to overtax a digestive system, especially if bed beckons within an hour or two; it takes around four hours for digestion to take place under optimal conditions, and much longer if the meal consists of meat and fat. Note that sleeping soundly on a full stomach hardly qualifies as optimal.

Nutritional Tenets of The Obvious Diet

Some of the central tenets of my own Obvious Diet come from the nutritional advice of my friend and client Dr. Mosaraf Ali, the famous healer and founder of the Integrated Medical Centre in London. In his wonderful and informative book *The Integrated Health Bible* (Vermilion, 2001) he offers these golden rules for losing weight:

1. Eat slowly.
2. Avoid acid foods.
3. Avoid alcohol.
4. Exercise regularly.
5. Avoid refined sugar, fatty or oily foods, and dairy products.

In general, Dr. Ali advocates avoidance of caffeine drinks, and instead an intake of at least six glasses of water per day, though he suggests limiting the consumption of fluids at mealtimes so as not to dilute the digestive juices. He also believes that dietary supplements should be treated with caution, as continuous use of powerful substances causes the body to become immune to the vitamin or mineral in question after a certain time. This is not to say that supplements don't have their place for people who are unable to digest food normally, are on a vegan diet, or for women who are pregnant or breast-feeding. Once again, though, medical advice is vital: some vitamins, for example, become toxic at high-enough doses.

A sample nutritionally balanced eating plan according to Dr. Ali looks something like this:

BREAKFAST Fruits, yogurt, and cereals, though protein such as eggs or cottage cheese are possible alternatives.

LUNCH The most substantial meal of the day, starting with a salad, then protein (fish or chicken), vegetables and carbohydrate (rice, yeast-free bread, potato, pasta, etc.). Any dessert should be eaten at least 45 minutes after the main course.

DINNER Unless eaten early, keep it light and avoid any foods that will not be digested fully by the time you go to bed (so no complex proteins such as red meat, or spicy food, either).

In addition, Dr. Ali advocates the setting aside of one day a week for what he calls a "Fasting Day," which in my diet I call a "Cleansing Day." This is such an integral part of The Obvious Diet that, as you will see, it has its own chapter. One day a week – I use Sundays because I am not involved in business breakfasts,

Dr. Ali advocates the setting aside of one day a week for a "Fasting Day."

One of the most important things you can do before embarking on The Obvious Diet is to pay a visit to a nutritionist.

lunches, or dinners where it might be difficult to practice abstinence – all I consume is juice, fruit, raw vegetables, and soup. The soup I have chosen is the (in)famous Cabbage Soup from the Cabbage Soup Diet (you will find the recipe for this soup in the Cleansing Day chapter). Why? Because many of my friends have tried this diet and averred that, yes, weight did come off as a result of using it. Also, I rather like the taste of it, probably because it reminds me of the delicious borscht my Russian-born mother used to make when I was a child (which was, however, full of the fatty juices of the flanken beef she used for the stock and was served with a large dollop of fattening sour cream!). I must admit that when I first contemplated a day off eating food as I knew it, I was full of apprehension. But actually it is an extremely pleasant experience. The soup is certainly filling, so no real hunger pangs are experienced and the end result is a feeling of lightness and well-being. The next day, I find I experience real hunger pangs, which, in the glutted world in which I live, is quite a rare experience.

Nutrition and Nutritionists

One of the most important things you can do before embarking on The Obvious Diet – something I would advise everybody to do if at all possible – is to pay a visit to a nutritionist. Not only are nutritionists/dietitians best placed to offer you general guidance on dietary rules, but they can help you find out if there are any foods you should absolutely avoid due to food intolerance or allergy. For many people a certain kind of food can throw the whole metabolic system out of phase. Strangely enough, these are often the foods we feel cravings for – for once, not an obvious idea. The effects of food intolerance vary widely and can resemble a whole litany of non-food-related problems. These can include eczema, bloating, water retention (extra weight), and feelings of weariness. The cure for food intolerance–related health problems is simplicity itself: the symptoms vanish when the offending food is removed from the diet. After a period of allergy-free living, it is often possible to reintroduce the food in question in small amounts.

You can contact the American Dietetic Association on the net at www.eatright.org. The site will help you find a nutritionist in your area.

Specific hypoallergenic diets are also available from a number of sources. These work by eliminating all the likely food intolerance culprits and then reintroducing them one by one.

Giving up is hard to do – there's no denying it.

One last suggestion for users of the Internet who are keen on finding nutritional advice is to consult the excellent resource maintained by the Tufts University Center on Nutrition Communication, which offers a vast number of rated links to nutritional and dietary sites.

In my case, as I have already said, when I first visited a nutritionist, I was told in no uncertain terms that I was averse to wheat, yeast, and gluten, which led to the banishment of bread, cereal, pasta, etc. from my diet. In addition, Dr. Ali completely banned cheese from my diet, a blow from which I am still trying to recover. It's not so much the bread I miss (although a good French baguette is hard to beat for a breakfast treat), but its animal-fat partners, butter and cheese. Giving up is hard to do – there's no denying it – but when the pounds start to fall away, you soon grasp the connection between your abstention and the body you want to have. Also, since I advocate a once-every-week treat, you can decide to eat whatever you want for one meal … and mine usually includes cheese!

All is not lost if you don't have the time, money, or inclination to make an appointment with a nutritionist. Elimination diets to discover food intolerances have been covered in great detail by many authors and often crop up in health magazines. Naturally, the Internet is an excellent source for finding out how other people rooted out the evil ingredient(s) in their diet – you can try typing in "elimination diet" to your favorite search engine and see what comes up.

I stress that professional help is by far preferable to the DIY approach; not even a plastic cup can be beyond suspicion, because cornstarch is used in its manufacture!

We keep our upper bodies in good shape by having a terrible fistfight every day (don't take that seriously, please).

Mel Brooks and Anne Bancroft

CHAPTER THREE

Getting Started

First things first: write everything down. Once you decide you want to embark on The Obvious Diet – your own unique weight reduction program, specially tailored to your own tastes and needs – get out your brand-new notebook and start making lists. The very act of putting in writing your desire to lose weight and your strategy for doing so is an important declaration of your serious intentions – the first shot you will fire in your Obvious Diet campaign.

To start the ball rolling, write down in your notebook exactly *why* you want to lose weight and how much you think you ought to lose. List on the left-hand side of a page what you think are the chief disadvantages of living with your present weight and your eating habits as they are. Then list on the right-hand side the flip side of the coin: the main advantages you think you stand to gain from losing weight and then keeping it off in the long run. Don't be put off by how "obvious" these lists look: the obvious often needs restating! Everybody's list will be different – obviously enough, as we all are different. My own list looked like this:

DISADVANTAGES

Don't like the look of my body.

I look/feel older with all this weight on me.

My clothes don't fit anymore.

Feel very heavy/sluggish after eating too much.

Disapprove/slightly ashamed of my own greediness.

I do not look or feel healthy.

ADVANTAGES

My body will look better.

I will look/feel younger.

My clothes will fit properly.

I will feel lighter, better.

I will be proud of my achievement.

I will look and feel healthy.

Through this initial list phase, you should keep (for a few days at least, and preferably a full week) a "diary" of *everything* you eat each day – and *why* you ate it. Take a two-page spread for each day of the week, and on the left-hand page write down the time of day, what you ate, and why. You may also want to note down whether you felt heavy and bloated or light and energized afterwards. It is a real eye-opener to see how much food you habitually eat without any thought whatsoever to its weight-producing potential or the amount you consume in total over the course of the day. There is a great deal of scope to reduce our intake of the needless, thoughtless snacks we habitually indulge in as markers in our daily lives, the reward food we eat whether or not we're hungry, and the oral gratification we seek at tough moments during the day.

A word on appetite might be appropriate at this point: there is a fundamental difference between appetite and hunger. Hunger is when the body needs food: your stomach starts to rumble and you're liable to want to eat something pretty soon. Appetite is another thing. It's when we're attracted to food, when the thought or sight or smell of some-thing gets the old juices going. If it's a craving, it gets us to make a beeline straight for the fridge/cookie jar/freezer. Precisely the kind of behavior The Obvious Diet seeks to overturn!

Next, make lists of the "dangerous" foods you already know put weight on you (you *do* know them!) and the "safe" foods you know are okay to eat without putting on the weight (you *do* know these too). My list was:

DANGEROUS FOODS

Bread and butter

Pasta

Mayonnaise

Bacon, sausage, and fatty meats

Fried foods

Fattening stews (e.g., cassoulet)

Heavy sauces

Nuts of all kinds (especially peanuts)

Beer/spirits

In general: avoid second and third helpings of all of the above!

SAFE FOODS

Fruits

Vegetables, raw and cooked

Fish of all kinds

Chicken

Grilled/steamed food

Lean meats

Olive oil, vinaigrette

Wine (in moderation!)

In general: eat less food!

Once again, I know all of this seems terribly obvious, but that is why the diet I am advocating actually works. It *is* obvious to you what you need to do in order to lose weight; what I am hoping to do is to help you connect with the knowledge you have already stored in your mind and the experience of the countless meals that have gone before to design a plan that will enable you to take (and keep!) the weight off and feel better about yourself.

Once you have kept up your food diary for a few days, on the right-hand page of your notebook you can start to write a parallel list of how you think you *should* be eating in an ideal world: less food in general and certainly less fattening food. "Should" is a big word, but what is important here is your own knowledge of yourself, the dictates of your conscience rather than some outside authority. Even as you look at the contrasting diaries of a day's actual eating versus a day of ideal eating, you can see how much lighter and better for you your nascent Obvious Diet plan looks.

While you are keeping your food diary is the ideal time to examine your personal dieting history. More lists! Write down lists of some of the diets you have already tried and discarded – you know, the ones you embarked upon with the highest of hopes and the best of intentions, before they became vague memories of past failures. What attracted you to these diets in the first place? What were the goals that you found easy to accomplish in the diets that you have tried?

What were the difficulties with those diets? You are trying to build up a profile of your own strengths and weaknesses in this area: what is easy for you to achieve; what is unfeasible. Bear in mind that what you are looking for in The Obvious Diet is the obvious solution: a plan for eating that helps you to feel better and lose weight *long-term*. You're putting together a personal plan that combines sound nutrition and weight-management principles and incorporates them into your own individual tastes and aptitudes.

The best way to do this is to browse through whatever diet books and articles you possess. If, like most people I know, you have built up your own collection from the huge number of published diet books, articles, and photocopies, you will soon be able to remind yourself of the principles that made sense to you. Since you are going to create your own Obvious Diet, you need not worry about slavishly following the precepts of these diets – all you want from them are the broad, general outlines that appeal to your own sense of how you can lose weight; and the ones that you know work for you but do not go

You should feel free to "mix and match" as many precepts from as many different diets as you wish.

against your daily living patterns, nor leave you feeling weak, tense, or irritable. For example, as you will see in Chapter Five, My Personal Eating Plan, I firmly believe that the "food combining" principles of the Hay Diet are very effective, and I incorporate its basic principles – do not mix proteins and carbohydrates in a single meal and eat fruit away from main meals – into my own Obvious Diet.

You should feel free to "mix and match" as many precepts from as many different diets as you wish; the only underlying rule is to design a plan you can follow effectively.

Well-Known Diets

As an aide-mémoire, here is an alphabetical list of well-known diets and a brief synopsis of the principles they espouse. Note that some of these diets may be known to you under other names – there's very little in the dieting world that hasn't been tried before. Note also that some of these diets are positively discouraged as long-term solutions by nutritionists because they lack vital nutrients and, in some cases, are based upon dubious underlying science. For example, popular high-protein, low-carbohydrate diets, a number of which are featured below, work on the nutritionally incorrect assumption that only carbohydrates, and not protein, can turn into fat. The reason people lose weight on these and indeed on any diet is because the diets restrict the total calorie intake. The golden rule of dieting, which can be extrapolated from all these diets, is that weight loss is achieved through taking in less energy (calories) than you expend.

Diets tend to fall into one of three categories: some ban or rely upon individual foods, some claim that certain foods have the ability to change the way the body handles food, while others still are based on the contention that specific hormones are the causes of all weight problems, and so elimination of those hormones leads to miracle weight loss. Single-food-based diets can shift weight, not so much because of the properties of the specific food concerned (grapefruit in the Grapefruit Diet, cabbage soup in the … you know that one already), but because repetitive consumption of the same food to the exclusion of others results in a depressed appetite which translates into less eating.

Atkins New Diet Revolution

This protein- and fat-rich diet promotes weight loss by severely limiting carbohydrate consumption. Although carbohydrates are gradually reintroduced by the end of the plan, they are below the almost 60 percent of total diet recommended by most nutritionists. The Atkins is perhaps the best-known of many high-protein/low-carbohydrate approaches to dieting and rapid weight loss. This and other high-protein/low-carbohydrate diets have been criticized because they can create a buildup of compounds called ketones, which are a threat to the kidneys and can produce unpleasant side effects such as bad breath.

Beverly Hills Diet

This is a 35-day plan starting with fruit only for the first ten days. Specific foods are added slowly and eaten at specific times during the day. Food combining is strongly discouraged, that is to say, avoidance of protein and carbohydrate consumption together. Some nutritionists, however, assert that the body actually processes food more effectively in combination.

Blood Type (Eat Right Diet)

Actually four differing diets for each of the four main blood group types, this diet is based on avoidance of specific foods. The (disputed) scientific theory is that each blood type is associated with a certain type of ancestral behavior, such as farming, nomadic life, and hunter/gathering, and that avoidance of certain types of food results in a lower incidence of disease.

Cabbage Soup Diet

This rapid-weight-loss regimen lasting one week is based on consumption of as much cabbage soup as you can eat, plus specific extras. It is also known as the "Sacred Heart Memorial Hospital 7 Day Fat Burning Diet," reputedly because it was invented at a medical center where coronary patients needed to lose weight fast. This, like other single-food diets, has been criticized for lacking balance.

Cambridge Diet

This rapid-weight-loss plan uses meal-substitute milk shakes and soups to supplement one regular balanced meal per day. Skipping a meal undoubtedly reduces overall daily calorie consumption, but many people find it hard to get through dips in blood sugar in the hours they are sustained only by the low-calorie drink. Also, if the body thinks that it is entering a time of starvation, it automatically slows down the metabolism to conserve supplies – making it harder, not easier, to shed weight.

Exchange Plans

As the basis of a number of commercial brand-name diet programs, foods are divided into categories such as carbohydrates, proteins, etc. for a long-term eating plan. In some versions foods are given a points rating, with a daily total for overall consumption. Any food within a certain group may be substituted for any other. These diets benefit from the motivational factor of being part of a community and sharing your support and experience with like-minded dieters.

Fit for Life

This food combination–based diet is built around high

consumption of fruit and vegetables.

Food Combining for Health

The theory behind this diet is to improve digestion by a regimen of never eating protein and carbohydrates together, low intake of high-fat dairy foods, and consumption of fruit away from meals. A number of popular diets, such as the Hay Diet, share this principle. Many people feel that this approach improves their digestion, but there have been criticisms that the omnivorous human body is designed to eat what it can get, when it can get it, without the niceties of worrying whether it's protein and carbohydrate at the same sitting.

F-plan

The more fiber (the F in the name) in the diet, the less time food and calories have to be absorbed by the body – or so the theory goes. As a bonus, fiber bulks out and fills up the stomach, reducing appetite. However, a sudden increase in the consumption of high-fiber foods can result in flatulence and gassiness.

Glucose Revolution

This diet counsels eating foods with a low glycemic index – every food has its rating – in order to keep blood sugar levels steady and reduce the body's production of insulin.

Grapefruit Diet

The theory here is that half a grapefruit before every meal provides fat-burning enzymes. Calorie intake is severely limited in this diet, which lasts up to three weeks, and as in other specific-food diets, the boredom factor has the twin effect of limiting food consumption and/or making it very difficult to stay the course.

Hip and Thigh Diet

An ultra-low-fat approach featuring high consumption of fruit, vegetables, and carbohydrate-rich foods. Calorie intake is kept low, and exercise is recommended to tackle problem areas of the body.

Juice-based diets

Fasting for variable numbers of days, with sustenance provided by pure fresh-squeezed fruit and vegetable juices, forms the basis of this very low-calorie diet. Some nutritionists have questioned the validity of fasting, despite its long tradition in certain cultures.

Low-fat diets

The use of low-fat or fat-free versions of pre-prepared foods as preferred to their high-fat equivalents is promoted in these diets, often without focusing on the nutritional balance of other elements in the diet. The pitfall here is that processed products in low-fat versions often replace the fat with high quantities of sugar or salt, which are either empty non-nourishing calories or could be a danger to people who suffer from diabetes and/or high blood pressure.

Mayo Clinic Diet

This low-carbohydrate plan is based on consuming as much meat as you can eat combined with the reputed slimming properties of grapefruit and a low intake of carbohydrates to lose weight.

Pritikin Diet

Originally developed as a diet for heart patients, this diet replaces processed foods and animal proteins with whole grains and vegetarian-oriented alternatives.

Scarsdale Diet

This long-standing favorite diet of many people begins with a two-week rigid low-calorie period that drastically limits carbo-hydrates in favor of unlimited lean protein. The initial phase is followed by a maintenance period that is intended to serve as training for healthy long-term eating. As in the case of other low-carbohydrate diets, nutritionists question the balance of food intake on this diet.

Sugar Busters Diet

The underlying principle here is that refined sugar is the enemy as it causes overproduction of insulin, which triggers extra storage of fat. Many foods are therefore eliminated, including simple carbohydrates, though complex, high-fiber carbohydrates are allowed. The scientific claims underpinning this diet have been called into question in some quarters.

System S Diet

The opposite of Sugar Busters, this diet actively encourages sugar consumption in the form of carbohydrates to keep blood sugar levels up as part of a calorie-controlled diet plan.

Zone Diet

The premise of this diet is that the optimum ratio of carbohydrate to protein to fat for burning the most calories is 40–30–30. This ratio is a long way outside the ratio nutritionists commonly recommend, (roughly) 60–20–20. Set meals with an exact calorie intake are, in effect, low-calorie, which promotes weight loss regardless of whether or not the science behind the diet is valid. Some dieters have had difficulty with the complicated tallies and calculations required to follow this diet.

My Dos and Don'ts

BANNED

Animal fat (butter, cheese)

Mushrooms, fungi in general
(Dr. Ali)

Lemon/other citrus (Dr. Ali)

Chicken skin (friend who
lost weight after bypass
operation)

Proteins/carbohydrates in
same meal (Hay Diet)

Bread

Pasta

Cereal

DISCOURAGED

Red/fatty meat (lamb,
beef, pork)

Dairy products (milk, yogurt,
ice cream)

WELCOMED

Fish

Lean meat

Fruit

Vegetables (especially
green veg.)

Juices

TOLERATED

Wine

Tea

Preparing Your Own Obvious Diet

So, having gathered the essential nutritional advice you need,
reviewed diets you have been on in the past that you could
contemplate revisiting in the future, and, preferably, found out

about any food intolerances and allergies you may have, you are ready to make a definitive list of dos and don'ts for your Obvious Diet. This is how mine looked (previous page).

Armed with this information, I went back to modify and refine my list of "dangerous" and "safe" foods that I drew up from my own lifetime store of information.

After finding out all the things you should and shouldn't be eating, it's time to see what you actually will be eating from now on. Now is the moment for the final (and probably most pleasant) part of preparing your Obvious Diet, as you sift through your favorite recipe books and find meals you would like to eat that fit in with the diet you are designing. This is a very happy task, for if you are like me, an enthusiastic eater, browsing through cookbooks is a wonderfully salivating experience, a gastronomic version of armchair travel! You will be surprised at how many of your favorite books contain recipes that are not only delicious, but follow more or less precisely the strictures of the diet program you are designing for yourself. Just because you can't eat the richest dishes in your most beloved cookbooks doesn't mean that you cannot enjoy other, less fattening delights you might otherwise have overlooked. Very often it is exceedingly easy to tweak recipes and make them much more healthy, for example, by not stirring all that cream into the sauce at the end, or by drastically reducing the amount of sugar that goes into a dessert. Because we usually stick to a surprisingly small number of recipes for our daily eating routines, it is important that you amass quite a list of dishes in your Obvious Diet notebook – just as it's important to vary the kinds of meals you eat, even though the basic precepts of what you are eating should be invariable. You can, of course, also use my own personal favorite recipes which I have included in this book (see pages 260–263 for a list) to get ideas.

So, now you have your knowledge of what constitutes a healthy, balanced diet for the average member of the human race, a list of foods you cannot – and, much more importantly, you can! – eat plus a list of recipes that conform to those restrictions. What's next? Actually getting started!

Choosing the Day to Start Your Obvious Diet

First of all, you need to pick a special day, be it the first day of the year, or a month, or your birthday, or the beginning of Lent or some other auspicious occasion. I know it seems a weakness of character to need such cajoling, but my experience of my own psyche – let alone those of my friends – leads me to believe that it is essential to build up to a target date for blastoff. It's hard to jump into a pool you know will be cold, and often dipping in a toe just has the effect of persuading you to walk rapidly in the opposite direction. Sometimes there's no other way than just to plunge in, and then you realize that, hey, the water's not so bad after all!

Next, it is very helpful to have a "sponsor" in this venture; someone who approves of, understands, and encourages the process you have embarked upon. In my case, it is my wife, Carol, who constantly nips at my heels to control my weight, and who is the person whose plaudits I seek for my weight loss. But it can be anybody you like: not just your partner but your doctor, a colleague at work, your children, or a friend. The involvement of other people is an essential component of your resolve to change your eating habits, not just for encouragement or approbation, but also because it provides a wider context for your efforts.

None of this is easy – I never claimed it was!

None of this is easy – I never claimed it was! – so you will need (and be grateful for) every bit of help you can get to start it and keep it going. A corollary to this is the fact that, once a group of people know you are doing your Obvious Diet, it becomes harder to quit ... or cheat ... and that is no bad thing!

Knowing Your Weak Spots

And now for your get-out-of-jail-free card – of no use now but handy to keep around for later in the game. Write down what it was that, in the past, brought your diet resolve to an end. It could have been a drunken moment, something that happened in your life that left you down and craving your favorite off-limits food, or a general lack of confidence in ever achieving the weight you want. See if you can spot a pattern to these events, especially immediately prior to the diet breaking down. If you can see a pattern, then you can also, hopefully, spot the symptoms of going off the rails before it's too late. Underline these

Write down what it was that, in the past, brought your diet resolve to an end.

symptoms in red pen, several times. Consign them to memory. And if, on your Obvious Dict, you should ever notice these symptoms occurring, you can pick them up in advance and neatly head them off. Because this time it's going to be different – this time you're fighting with, not against yourself.

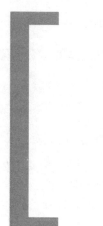

**Never eat when
you're not hungry,
no matter how
impolite you feel.**

Ken Follett

CHAPTER FOUR

The First Month

What you should have after all that work is your set of Obvious rules you think will work for you to keep your weight in check, provide you with the necessary nutrients you need to do what you do, and fit in with your lifestyle. You should have a set of recipes that adhere to these guidelines, which you may or may not have arranged into a meal-by-meal plan, or you may prefer to keep as a stock cupboard into which you can dip as required – the approach you take depends entirely on which method feels best for you.

But The Obvious Diet is not all laissez-faire, especially in the first month. There are some "first principles" which I feel to be important.

Kick-starting The Obvious Diet is the only way to begin, because old habits die hard. When you think about it, among the very few things in our daily lives over which we have absolute control are how much and what we eat and how much and what kind of exercise we take. The very fact that you are reading this book means that you are concerned about your body and aware that getting rid of excess weight and being physically active are major factors in ensuring a long, healthy, happy life. We all know this; it is totally obvious!

Our eating habits are just that: deeply ingrained, long-term patterns of behavior. But we know that habits – even addictions – are capable of being overturned permanently with a few weeks' concerted effort. Embarking on a major change in my

Kick-starting The Obvious Diet is the only way to begin, because old habits die hard.

eating patterns was, for me, very much like giving up cigarettes. The analogy is perfect, because in both cases it's a question of absolutely shifting your whole way of being – suddenly and not gradually, or the addiction will never be conquered. I gave up smoking on May 1, 1976, at 2:00 p.m. at the London Tara Hotel in Kensington; the precision of that memory ought to give you an indication of how important a moment that was for me! Until then, I had smoked two packs a day for twenty years from the age of sixteen. But somewhere along the way – perhaps spurred on by my children who kept complaining about my smoking – my concerns about the health hazards smoking posed finally became more important to me than feeding my habit.

Smoking cigarettes and eating too much of the wrong

kinds of food have a lot in common. We know perfectly well we shouldn't be doing them (the smoker's hacking cough, the overindulgent eater's feeling of heaviness and surplus weight provide vivid evidence of the errors of our ways), but the infantile urge for oral gratification overpowers adult common sense

Smoking and eating too much of the wrong kinds of food have a lot in common.

and we continue to eat or smoke ourselves into crisis. The tipping point occurs when you fully grasp and truly accept that the rewards of modifying your behavior outweigh the rewards of indulging.

I grew up in a large Jewish family in New York where food was, literally, love, and where the cliché "Eat, eat, it's good for you" was a daily refrain. My memories of my early eating life are of huge quantities of fatty foods – chopped liver oozing with chicken fat, slice upon slice of pot-roasted brisket of beef, and vast deli sandwiches – in an endless procession of family meals at home or in restaurants. Eating two or three portions was considered a polite (and obligatory!) compliment to my mother's cooking abilities, and, to this day, I still have an overpowering urge to eat far more than I know is necessary or desirable. When the message came through that enough was enough, that my hunger was satisfied, I simply ignored it and demolished whatever remained in the path of Hurricane Ed.

Because overeating is a form of addiction – and we know that, in any addiction situation, "the devil never sleeps" – I believe the transition from the bad old ways to the sensible and healthy approach to eating we wish to achieve needs to be absolute. Cutting down is still playing the game. The quicker you instill discipline into your eating patterns, the more immediate – and therefore gratifying! – the rewards will be. That is why the first month of your Obvious Diet should be as rigorous as possible.

You may well ask at this point how does this stern approach differ from other strict diets? The answer is, once again, obvious: of your own volition you are adhering to a set of dietary restrictions that you have set up for yourself and that you – and you alone! – are responsible for establishing and administering. There is no fascistic menu prescription: "it's Wednesday morning so you must eat yogurt and bananas" despite the fact that you may not have either yogurt or bananas in the house. There are no must-eat food combinations, no complex points systems to learn, no demonized foods – unless you have specifically decided that this is the best way for you to achieve your long-term Obvious Diet eating plan. Under The Obvious Diet, you have a great deal of choice

Cutting down is still playing the game.

in the specific foods you eat, as long as they adhere to the general dietary purposes you have set up for yourself. The first month of The Obvious Diet is like an airplane flight: a slight, relatively brief period of discomfort which is well worth the benefit of arriving at a new place. If you aren't prepared to fly, your horizons are always going to look like they do now.

The first month is about breaking old habits, and you can rest assured that much of what we believe to be inalienable truths about ourselves, our likes and dislikes, and possibilities, is no more than deeply ingrained habit, the furrow left by a pattern repeated over and over again. We are all capable of so much more.

So, the first month is transition. The difference between the first month of your Obvious Diet and your long-term eating plan (I will outline mine in detail in the next chapter – see page 79 – as an example of how one man's Obvious Diet looks) is TOTAL abstinence from the stuff you know is bad for you. I am afraid this includes the elimination of all alcohol, all sugar, all fatty foods – the things you already know put weight on you. In my own case, during this month I also decided to go without any red meat, which I found to my great surprise, as a lifelong carnivore, I hardly missed at all. I mainly confined my first-course eating to salads and my main-course eating to fish and chicken (with the skin always removed, of course!).

Anyone who knows me knows that I am the last person in the world you would expect to preach abstinence.

The adjective that has most often accompanied my name in the press is "flamboyant." All I am preaching – I can hear my voice and to my surprise I *am* preaching here – is the *modulation* (not elimination!) of your desires. A piece of plain grilled fish, drizzled with olive oil and scattered with herbs, may not be a medium rare 16-ounce prime New York sirloin steak with fries ... but it certainly tastes wonderful in itself. I am not saying you must follow my example in cutting out red meat during the first month; if you do want to eat red meat, just make sure it is as lean as possible (veal is probably the best choice).

Anyone who knows me knows that I am the last person in the world you would expect to preach abstinence.

Maybe it's something else that you have to steer clear of during the first month, but whatever the food item is that turns you on, whatever has in the past been the high point of your meal, the item that made you salivate, the thing that shouted loudest at you from the restaurant menu, if it's on your list of proscribed foods, this is the time to break the Pavlovian reaction. For what? you may quite rightly ask. To be amazed at how good and how light you feel after a few days following your new regime.

Alcohol

The giving up of alcohol is a vexed subject for most people – myself included. I am convinced that it is essential to cut it out for the first month, just as much to establish discipline as to minimize your intake of calories.

I confess I love to drink wine and have a wonderful collection of it, which I will never, ever permanently forsake. Oddly enough, though, I have never had a problem giving up drinking for a month a year. In fact, for the past fifteen years, I have established the ritual of an "alcohol-free August" – perhaps the precursor to my conviction that the first month of my Obvious Diet should be as absolute as possible. This originally came about because my two older sons, Adam and Ivan, who had already hounded me about those cigarettes, took me aside one summer's day at our Bridgehampton home and, with a serious look on their faces, started lecturing me on how they thought I

Giving up actually turned out to be far easier than I expected.

was drinking too much. I didn't agree with them at all, but the more I thought about it, the more I began to worry that they might be right. So, I decided to give up drink for one month on August first and resume on September first. Giving up actually turned out to be far easier than I expected. Yes, I had to renounce what until then had been a pleasure I took for granted, but there were other things I gained in recompense: for example, instead of feeling drowsy after our evening meal, I was bright and wide awake, often reading for hours into the night, something I could never do after imbibing. There was also a certain amount of weight loss simply as a result of cutting out alcohol – without any other appetite restrictions or modifications. In fact, the whole experiment was so successful that I decided to make every August an "alcohol-free zone" – a ritual I have followed religiously for many, many years.

Sugar

Sugar is another major problem area. You don't need me to tell you that the cravings of a sugar-fiend are quite as strong as those of a smoker or drinker for their particular weakness. Again it is important to establish an initial underlying discipline before relaxing into a long-term healthy-eating plan that allows you the occasional splurge. We're talking about a month here, not forever. It's not as if you've had your last ever taste of tiramisu or cake. Somehow the taste for sweets was left out of my system, so it is easy for me to say no to desserts or choco-late or ice cream. But I am married to an inveterate sweet eater who gives me the following hint for anyone who cannot entirely deny his sweet tooth. This I share with you now, though strictly speaking I advocate sticking to

You should try as hard as you can to "stay hungry."

the letter of your newly created law for the first month: she believes that dark chocolate containing 60 percent or more cocoa can be eaten without weight gain, and within a couple of weeks it is just as satisfying a treat as any gooey dessert.

Enough's Enough

Another important aspect of the first month's dieting is the actual amount you eat.

You should try as hard as you can to "stay hungry." There really is nothing more obvious than the fact that eating less is necessary to reduce weight, and so it is for the vast majority of people. Instead of ordering two courses at a restaurant, try ordering just a main course or two appetizers.

Healthy Snacks

Whether at home or in a restaurant, *always leave some food on your plate* – you don't need to eat it all. What happens if you are still hungry? Some people are hungry always, regardless of how recently they last ate and how much they have polished off. Hunger comes in multiple flavors. There's the food we physiologically need to consume for our body to function, and then there's all the rest: the delicacies we just can't turn down when they pass

> **Whether at home or in a restaurant, *always leave some food on your plate*.**

under our noses, the reward food we promise ourselves for getting through the next hour, the careless snacks we chomp without even noticing in front of the television, the food we eat as markers of time at certain points during the day, the comfort food we've just got to have when the world seems to be a hostile place....

The key is to think about *why* you want to eat in a given situation, to make it a conscious action rather than just an unthinking habit. Do you always want to reach for something sweet in the middle of the afternoon when your energy has slumped? Go for a quick walk around the block and revive yourself with some fresh air instead. Do you get home from work and head straight for a glass of wine or vodka and tonic? Instead have a bath or shower to wash away the accumulated stress and make sure you feel more relaxed before you approach the fridge or liquor cabinet. Question yourself – are you really hungry or is it just an emotional need? If you decide you really are genuinely hungry you can take pleasure in satisfying that need and know you are not simply falling into an automatic pattern.

It is, in general, better to have more frequent, small meals instead of one or two large ones. A lifesaver – a diet-saver at

> **It is, in general, better to have more frequent, small meals instead of one or two large ones.**

A lifesaver is always to have some healthy snacks on hand.

least – is always to have some healthy snacks on hand, especially if you are the kind of person whose blood sugar levels can suddenly drop. The best snacks for such moments, to my mind, are a supply of fresh, raw vegetables. Before I went on The Obvious Diet I used to love coming home from work – on those evenings when I was not going straight from my office to a cocktail party or have drinks with friends – and devouring chunks of ham. Not gourmet Parma ham or fancy hand-carved baked ham but those chunks sold off cheap at my grocer because no one else wanted them – the odd bits and pieces from near the bone, full of fat, skin, and gristle. To tell the absolute truth, they were bought for our Yorkshire terrier, Pepsi, who, lacking the opposable thumbs to get to the fridge first, had to share them with her greedy human. Now, I have found the perfect evening snack to fit in with my Obvious Diet. It is a simple, delicious recipe for Vegetables in Mustard Vinalgrette from *The Martha Stewart Cookbook* (see Chapter Six, Living with The Obvious Diet). Same hour, same craving, same satisfaction. No, actually, a greater satisfaction in feeling good that I can so easily fulfill my snack craving yet remain within the borders of my Obvious Diet!

The Cleansing Day

During the first month the Cleansing Day must be very strictly observed, because it will establish the habit for the long run. But, alas, I do not recommend that the Treat Meal – when you get to eat whatever your appetite desires – should start until after the first month has been completed. The Treat Meal is reserved for those who make it through the transitional phase and it's the reward for doing so well. This does not mean that one slip from the path you have mapped out for yourself is a disaster. It's the long haul that counts, the journey to a better, healthier relationship with food. If things get dangerously depressing, it is obviously better for you to have the occasional drink or dessert rather than feel defeated. If you must, satisfy the craving, then move on, what's done is done. You must be the judge, which in the first month means showing leniency on yourself in the face of mitigating circumstances.

Exercise

As you can see, the first month is essential to establish a routine for your eating. It is also the ideal opportunity to establish a routine for your personal exercise. Exercise really is an essential part of The Obvious Diet. Burning more calories than in the past is key to losing weight. But exercise does more than just burn off excess fat: it improves your general strength, it gives you a sense of achievement, and it makes you feel good because it releases endorphins. It is also a way of venting the tensions and stresses that inevitably build up.

My personal exercise regime is a one-hour mixture of stretching, aerobics, and weight training every Monday, Wednesday, and Friday before breakfast. I usually start between 7:00–7:30 a.m., so that I am not interrupted by the steady stream of phone calls that begins coming in at home from 8:30 onward (many of my clients, like me, start their day early!). The first part of my routine is a fairly complete set of stretches. I concentrate on stretching all the big muscle groups – legs, arms, and abdomen. I also do a few basic yoga postures, which I find helps to clear my mind for the new day ahead. This takes around twenty minutes. Then I switch to aerobics. Using a Reebok step, I do 200 steps in all, quite enough to raise my heartbeat and respiration to the required degree. These are broken down as 50 steps on the right leg (followed by 30 squats), 50 steps on the left leg (followed by 30 squats), 50 steps on the right leg again (followed by 30 push-ups), and finally 50 steps on the left leg again. I then do a set of abdominal exercises for about 5 minutes, followed by a few more stretches on the floor. The final part of my routine is weight training. I use both dumbbells and barbells, and take great care not to injure my back (using an exercise belt is essential). I do presses, curls, flies, etc. for about twenty more minutes, making a total of about an hour. I finish off with a few final stretches. (Once, many years ago, I struck up a conversation on an airplane with someone who had been the physical trainer for the New York Giants, who explained to me that the single most important part of any exercise routine is stretching.)

Exercise works in so many ways: expending energy makes you feel better, it helps you tone up, and it is a concrete measure of how much fitter you are becoming – far more reaffirming than those banished scales. But, as with everything in The Obvious Diet, your exercise program can be exactly what you want it to be, tailored to fit in with your life, as long as you put in the minimum requirement of three times a week. And if you can't exercise at the regular times you have set aside for the purpose, don't worry; find another time to fit it in. Please remember that people who tend to lead sedentary lives and are not used to taking exercise are always encouraged to seek advice from a doctor or trainer before beginning an exercise program, as sudden furious physical activity after a long period of inactivity is an almost sure-fire path to injury.

As with everything in The Obvious Diet, your exercise program can be exactly what you want it to be.

Do not expect any miracles in the first couple of weeks; it will take at least four weeks – and quite possibly more – for you to start noticing weight peel away. But it will happen! And it will happen sooner the more strictly you adhere to the first month of totally disciplined eating. Besides the huge reward of seeing your old body shape reemerge, what will happen, and this I guarantee, is that you will feel 100 percent better within yourself and about yourself.

What I have outlined above is my own "kick-start" to The Obvious Diet – the ways and means I used to achieve my initial weight loss. You may ask yourself at this point: how is The Obvious Diet different from "crash diets" you have seen and perhaps tried in the past? Well, at this stage of the game, it isn't really very different because, like most diets, The Obvious Diet advocates tough tactics to initiate the weight loss process. Where it does greatly differ from most diets is that the most important part of this whole approach is the *long-term process*, the way you can keep your body weight where you want it to be while leading your usual life. If any of the other diets I outlined seems to offer a more effective weight loss regime in your particular case, use it, incorporate it into your plan. Remember, you're the one making the rules here. You know in your heart of hearts what's most likely to work for you, and that's what you're trying to achieve.

Summer diet: time to pin the rules on the fridge door. Anything you drink, apart from water, is food.

Koo Stark

CHAPTER FIVE

My Personal Eating Plan

Having given you in Chapters Two and Three general principles on how to set about designing your personal eating plan, I would now like to describe to you in detail my own plan, so you can hopefully learn from my example. I want to emphasize – yet again – that the central tenet of The Obvious Diet is that *only the diet you design for yourself* will give you the results that you desire and deserve. So, as you read through my plan, you should be simultaneously thinking about the shape of your own plan to meet your individual needs.

You will remember that my visit to the nutritionist revealed certain foods that I needed to avoid absolutely – among them, wheat, gluten, and yeast. Therefore any eating plan I created for myself would have to take account of these banished foods. Also, as you may recall, I decided to try to avoid red meat during the first month ... a principle that very easily transferred itself to my long-term Obvious Diet, although modified to being a radical reduction rather than a total prohibition. So, as I planned my diet, I tended to concentrate on fish and chicken as the main-course elements of a diet that stressed both raw and cooked vegetables plus lots of fresh fruit. I also mentioned the fact that I believed in the principles of food combining, as set out in the Hay Diet. This is because, at one point in my life, I went on the Hay Diet and found myself painlessly losing weight – not quickly, but over a period of months, before eventually, as with all the diets I tried before I embraced The Obvious Diet, I "fell off the wagon" and abandoned the very principles that had served me so well.

The central tenet of The Obvious Diet is that *only the diet you design for yourself* will give you the results that you desire and deserve.

As you will have gathered from the summary of diets in Chapter Three, the classic Food Combining Diet is very easy to follow. Although it has its detractors, who allege that there is absolutely no scientific basis for its claims, I can personally vouch for its efficacy as a weight-reducing regime. Its central thesis is that, in order to maximize the absorption of the nutrients in the food we eat, we should not mix proteins (such as meat, poultry, fish, or eggs) with carbohydrates (such as potatoes, pasta, rice, or bread) in the same meal, because the digestive processes of those two food groups are entirely different. Also to be avoided is mixing different types of protein, for example, meat and dairy. Fruit must be eaten only on its own, and never added to a regular meal. Vegetables combine with either proteins or carbohydrates or can be eaten on their own with no digestive problems. To round things off, the Hay Diet, and other versions of the food combining approach to eating, offers a list of foods that are best avoided in general. These range from items containing refined sugars and refined flour to pork products, peanuts, and coffee. I find it interesting how many of these "enemies" crop up in different diets as demonized foods. Consumption of processed foods and items rich in highly refined foods is, food scientists never seem to tire telling us, a prime reason why over the last few decades people in the West have reduced their overall calorie intake but more and more often suffer from obesity.

My general goal was very, very simple: to (a) eat less and (b) eat better.

My general goal was very, very simple: to (a) eat less and (b) eat better. So, to start the day, I try to have only fruit salad. No eggs, no bacon, sausage, or other breakfast meats, no cereal, and no milk. My daily breakfast usually consists of a mixture of strawberries and raspberries, which, I was advised by a doctor friend, constitute something of an anti-cancer diet. But I am also happy to have bananas, grapes, papaya, mango ... or just a general mélange of fruit. Because of Dr. Ali's prohibition of citrus fruit, I tend to avoid oranges and grapefruit in fruit salad. Sometimes I mix a little live low-fat yogurt into my fruit, but, in general, I try to avoid too much dairy produce, so my brushes with yogurt are relatively rare. If I haven't got time to sit down and eat my fruit salad, I'll grab a banana and eat it on the way to work or the golf course. A banana makes a convenient – and delicious – breakfast on the run, and provides an immediate energy boost to start the day. Beginning each day with fruit salad makes that hectic moment of the day so much easier – no choice and very little work, especially if you make a large bowl of fruit salad that can last out the week in the fridge.

You may prefer to get things moving each morning with eggs or cereal with skimmed milk or yogurt, for example, depending on your individual taste and nutritional require-ments. One thing I would say is that sticking with the same breakfast, more or less day after day, ensures no deviation from your regime in the mornings and makes a start that helps set the tone for the rest of the day's eating. If I want to have eggs – my client Freddie Forsyth and his wife, Sandy, live on a farm in Hertfordshire and regularly send us the best, freshest eggs, which are irresistible! – I try to have them boiled or poached, the least fattening way to eat them. But if, every now and then, you want to have some scrambled eggs, please go very easy on the butter, using just the minimum to make sure the eggs don't stick to the pan. Another breakfast treat which will not interfere with your diet is smoked fish. If waking up to a hotel buffet in a foreign city (which happens to me all too often!), I sometimes treat myself to a small portion of smoked fish – smoked salmon is an elegant, delicious, and relatively non-fattening breakfast food. You could also have smoked mackerel, halibut, or sturgeon – indeed any other smoked fish. As with any meal on The Obvious Diet, try not to eat too much of these good things, although it is true that eating a proper breakfast is a healthy way to begin your day.

Once again, as I was spared a sweet-tooth gene in my makeup, I am fortunate in not having to fight the morning lure of sugar. One tactic for people whose constitution cries out for a sweet rather than savory start to the day is to convert to high-fruit spreads, where the sweetening element is grape-juice concentrate. My Italian daughter-in-law, Patrizia, I know, is very partial to a breakfast of one of these "jams" (though they're made up of pure fruit, they cannot legally call themselves jams in the U.K. precisely

> **I was spared a sweet-tooth gene in my makeup.**

because they aren't stuffed full of sugar!) spread over a layer of ricotta, on whole wheat bread.

Everybody has their favorite breakfast drink, and usually this part of the meal will not present a weight risk – except if you load too much sugar into your tea or coffee! I tend to use sugar substitute – which, it could be argued, is not in itself a very healthy option. But, given the choice of eating sugar or a sugar substitute, I, like many other people, will go for the sub- stitute nine times out of ten because of the calorie issues involved. Of course, you would be much better off drinking only herbal teas rather than the usual cups of caffeine, but life does need a few pleasures, and caffeine is the one that I have decided to indulge in (without overindulging!). Incidentally, a truly healthy way to start the day is to sip some hot water – with or without lemon – before you take in any other breakfast drink.

All dieters have to make personal sacrifices, and the traditional cooked breakfast has been one of my biggest.

My habitual morning drink is English Breakfast tea, which I take with skimmed milk and that sugar substitute. Coffee went out of my life three years ago, when, lurching towards

Frankfurt airport in the back of a big, old Mercedes taxicab one Sunday morning after the annual Frankfurt Book Fair, I felt so sick from the endless cups of morning coffee I had consumed that I almost lost the will to live! After that cab ride I never had a cup of coffee again!

As for juices, since my diet prohibits citrus, I try to avoid the typical glass of orange or grapefruit juice, and content myself with a glass of apple or cranberry juice. If you happen to have a juicer – and I highly recommend that if you don't, you acquire one soon – it is fun and delicious; a cocktail of fresh fruit juices forms an excellent part of any Obvious Diet. My own favorite combination is apple, papaya, and strawberry – but, once you have a juicer in your kitchen, you can experiment to your heart's content.

You will, no doubt, have noticed that breakfast meats are conspicuously absent from my menus – and should be from yours. All dieters have to make personal sacrifices, and this has been one of my biggest. The traditional bacon, sausage, and egg breakfast (the term "fry-up" speaks all too eloquently for itself in this context!) is, I freely admit, a delicious institution (and one that I do sometimes choose for my Treat Meal). But it is also, of course, very heavy and fatty – a bloating and weight-inducing

Try to stick either to one course or two appetizers.

way to begin your day. Not so bad, perhaps, if you habitually spend the morning working it off on a construction site, but a heart-stopping start for the majority of us whose journey to work is followed by hours in a chair. As I have said, The Obvious Diet is about changing your expectations about what constitutes a satisfying meal. And, once you relegate the traditional cooked breakfast, or whatever morning misdemeanors you previously indulged in, to an occasional treat and substitute a much lighter, healthier alternative, you will soon be more than satisfied with your new way of starting your day's food account.

The Obvious Diet is about changing your expectations about what constitutes a satisfying meal.

My lunches and dinners consist generally of chicken or fish plus vegetables. I tend to eat out at lunchtime, so I carefully choose restaurants where I know I can order plain grilled chicken or fish and freshly cooked vegetables or salads. (See Chapter Six – Living with The Obvious Diet – for specific hints about how to keep to The Obvious Diet in restaurants.) As I mentioned earlier, the single most obvious point of The Obvious Diet is to eat less! To that end, you should always make it a practice to leave some food on your plate. Also, you should try to stick either to one course or two appetizers.

It is truly amazing how quickly your body will become acclimatized to your reduced intake of food. And no wonder! How often have you thought (as I certainly did!) that, by the time you finished your first course, you really had consumed enough food? But of course you went ahead and polished off the next course because you had ordered it anyway, and after breaking through the satiety barrier, you thought you just might as well continue to eat and eat – after all, the damage was done and all discipline long gone.

My Favorite Recipes

Although I am decidedly not – and never will be – a vegetarian, salads and simply cooked vegetables have now become the mainstay of my eating life on The Obvious Diet. As often as I can, I try to have meals without the central element of chicken or fish ... i.e., just salads or a plate of steamed or grilled vegetables. If you had stopped me in the street before I went on my new regime and told me I would be happy and sated with these kinds of meals, I would have laughed out loud. But, happily for us, just as old habits die hard, new habits are quick to form. Among the best recipes I know for delicious vegetable dishes are the following three from Ruth Gray and Ruth Rogers's cookbooks:

Marinated Grilled Vegetables

Cut the eggplant lengthwise into eighths and place in a colander with some sea salt. Cut the zucchini lengthwise into sixths or eighths depending on size, add some salt, and place in a separate colander. Leave both to drain of any bitter juices for a minimum of 30 minutes. Rinse and dry well.

Cut the peeled peppers into sixths, and place on a dish.

Place the eggplant and zucchini pieces on the hottest part of the grill and grill on both sides, seasoning at the same time with salt and pepper. The eggplant in particular requires care – it needs to be cooked, but should not be allowed to burn. To test, gently press with a finger; if it resists, it is not done. When it is cooked, keep separate from the zucchini.

Mix the olive oil with the lemon juice and garlic, and pour over the individual vegetables, gently lifting to coat them. Combine all the seasoned vegetables in a large bowl with the basil or marjoram leaves, turn over once, and taste for seasoning – it should be robust.

Serves 6

1 lb eggplant

1 lb zucchini

1 lb each of red and yellow peppers, seeded and peeled

sea salt and freshly ground black pepper

extra virgin olive oil (up to 7 oz)

juice of 2 lemons

2 garlic cloves, peeled and crushed in a little sea salt

a handful of fresh basil or marjoram

Roasted Asparagus

Serves 6

3 1/2 lb asparagus

olive oil

1 bunch fresh basil,
leaves picked from their
stems, roughly chopped

sea salt and freshly
ground black pepper

1 garlic clove, peeled
and finely chopped

4 oz Niçoise or calamata
olives, pitted

Preheat the oven to 425°F.

Trim the asparagus of any woody portion by gently flexing the base of the stem until it snaps. Discard the woody ends, and wash the green stalks and tips. Dry well and place in a mixing bowl. Toss with enough olive oil to lightly coat each stalk. Add the basil, salt, pepper, and garlic, and gently mix.

Arrange in an oiled roasting pan and season again. Add the olives.

Roast in the preheated oven for about 20 minutes or until the stalks are wilted and light gold in color.

(*Note* I prefer to roast the asparagus for 40 minutes to give them a browner, more "burnt" look and taste. But try it both ways – or somewhere in between – to suit yourself.)

Roasted Cherry Vine Tomatoes

Preheat the oven to 425°F.

Place the tomatoes in an oiled roasting pan. Sprinkle with the thyme and the garlic. Drizzle with oil, and season. Roast for 20 minutes.

(*Note* I prefer the look and taste of the tomatoes when roasted longer – anything up to one hour.)

Serves 6

3 ¼ lb cherry tomatoes, on the vine, in about 10 small clusters

3 tablespoons olive oil

1 bunch fresh thyme in small sprigs

3 garlic cloves, peeled and thinly sliced

sea salt and freshly ground black pepper

All of these recipes are easy to make, wonderful to eat, and store conveniently in the fridge for use later on, either re-heated or at room temperature.

There are, of course, literally thousands of ways to cook chicken and fish. But, like most people, I tend to stick to a few tried and trusted recipes. Of all the roast chicken recipes in the world, there are only two that I use regularly.

The first is one that is totally in keeping with my Obvious Diet, a recipe for Vertical Roast Chicken from the cookbook *Le Dome at Home*. This is one of the signature dishes from Le Dome, one of the most fashionable restaurants in Los Angeles, which caters to many celebrities and movie stars who watch what they eat with eagle eyes. Apart from being an utterly delicious method of cooking chicken, it is a perfect way to keep to your diet because all the fat runs off into the roasting pan, leaving only lean, moist meat to be served on a bed of mixed salad. As Eddie Kerkhofs, the talented Belgian proprietor of Le Dome, says in his prefatory remarks to the recipe: "This dish is very popular at my restaurant because there is no oil or butter in the preparation, yet it is moist and tender. There is no need to baste the chicken because the skin is dry and seals in the juices. Actually, the fat is the only thing that drips out, giving its flavor to the stock, which in turn evaporates back up into the chicken, returning all the flavor of the juices."

Vertical Roast Chicken on a Bed of Mixed Greens

Preheat the oven to 425°F.

Mix the chopped onion, shallot, tarragon, salt, pepper, and cayenne in a bowl. Set aside. This mixture is to be inserted between the skin and the meat of the chicken. In order to do this the skin must be loosened. Start by massaging the chickens gently; do not be too rough or you will damage the skin. Gently work your fingers between the skin and meat of the breasts and thighs until you have created a space. Be careful not to puncture the skin.

Once the skin is separated from the meat, place the seasoning mixture under the skin. In a 3-inch-deep roasting pan, place the chickens on two vertical roasters and arrange them so that they are approximately 2 inches apart.

Then, in a separate pan, bring the chicken stock to the boil and pour it into the bottom of the roasting pan. Place the pan in the oven.

Cook at this high heat for 20 minutes, then lower the heat to 375°F and cook for another 30 to 40 minutes without

1 medium white onion, chopped

1 medium shallot, chopped

1 tablespoon chopped fresh tarragon

$1/8$ teaspoon salt

$1/8$ teaspoon pepper

$1/8$ teaspoon cayenne pepper

2 2-lb whole chickens

2 cups chicken stock

2 heads Boston lettuce

1 head frisée (curly endive)

2 Belgian endive, washed and cut into 3-inch pieces

$1/2$ head Romaine lettuce, washed and cut into 3-inch pieces

$1/2$ cup vinaigrette dressing

basting. The chickens are done when the juices run clear. Remove them from the oven and let them stand on the roasters for 5 minutes.

Break the Boston lettuce and the frisée into pieces and put them both into a mixing bowl. Add the endive and the Romaine, pour in the vinaigrette, and toss. Spread the greens over the bottom of a large serving platter.

Remove the chickens from the roasting pan, leaving them on their vertical roasters. Carve off pieces of chicken with a small knife. The meat should separate from the bone very easily. Arrange the pieces of meat over the bed of greens and serve.

(Note You don't need to use two small chickens; one large one will do, and of course you can adjust the cooking time to accommodate this. And if you have trouble finding a "vertical roaster," you can do so on the Internet at many sites that sell kitchen goods.)

The second recipe is, to my mind, the single best recipe for roast chicken I have ever come across: Simon Hopkinson's great version in *Roast Chicken and Other Stories*. It does, of course, use butter, so there is an element of "cheating" here. But The Obvious Diet should never be regarded as an exact science – its virtue is that your Obvious Diet, which you have designed bearing in mind your personal likes and nutritional needs and lifestyle, is flexible enough to adapt to your commitments and to the occasional, shall we say, diversion without jeopardizing the long-term plan. There are obvious ways to make this more dietetic: substitute olive oil for butter, don't slosh the pan drippings over your chicken (and hopefully have the inner strength to remove the delicious skin), and it can fit in tolerably well to your overall plan. Here it is:

Roast Chicken

Preheat the oven to 450°F.

Smear the butter (or virtuous olive oil) with your hands all over the bird. Put the chicken in a roasting pan that will accommodate it with room to spare. Season liberally with salt and pepper and squeeze over the juice of the lemon. Put the herbs and garlic inside the cavity, together with the squeezed-out lemon halves – this will add a

1 stick butter, at room temperature

4-lb free-range chicken

salt and pepper

1 lemon

several sprigs of thyme or tarragon, or a mixture of the two

1 garlic clove, peeled and crushed

fragrant lemony flavor to the finished dish.

Roast the chicken in the oven for 10 to 15 minutes. Baste, then turn the oven temperature down to 375°F and roast for a further 30 to 45 minutes with further occasional basting. The bird should be golden brown all over with a crisp skin and have buttery, lemony juices of a nut-brown color in the bottom of the pan.

Turn off the oven, leaving the door ajar, and leave the chicken to rest for at least 15 minutes before carving. This enables the flesh to relax gently, retaining the juices in the meat and ensuring easy, trouble-free carving and a moist bird.

(*Note* You may remember that Dr. Ali banned lemons and lemon juice from my diet, so I eliminate the lemon from this recipe, with absolutely no diminution of pleasure from the final result.)

With either of these recipes, The Obvious Dieter – at least this Obvious Dieter – has a difficult choice at the table: to eat the skin or not to eat the skin. Clearly, the skin from the Vertical Roast Chicken is less of a problem because, theoretically, the fatty layer just under the skin has melted and run down into the pan. The skin on Simon Hopkinson's bird is, however, another story, and there your conscience needs to be your guide.

Another very simple and dietetic way to eat chicken (which eliminates the skin conundrum) is simply to grill a chicken paillard (this is a boneless, skinless chicken breast which has been pounded very flat by the butcher) brushed with olive oil and herbs of your choice (I like rosemary). Despite the French name, these chicken breasts are generally served in Italian homes too; I may be wrong, but I suspect that any culinary staple that the French and Italians agree on must have something going for it! It cooks (grilling or poaching in water or stock) in a couple of minutes, and, served on top of a mixed green salad with vinaigrette dressing, makes a tasty but extremely light meal.

Grilled Paillards

2 chicken paillards
olive oil
fresh herbs, such as
rosemary, thyme, or
cilantro

Brush the paillards with the olive oil and press the herbs (you can use any or all of the herbs at your disposal) into the flesh.

Grill for two minutes per side under a very hot broiler or cook on a very hot grill pan on top of the stove. Outside, the paillards should be a crispy golden color, and inside the flesh should be moist and delicious.

(*Note* It is a good idea to order several of these paillards from your butcher and keep a supply of them, individually wrapped, in your freezer. They thaw and cook very quickly, and make a perfect light meal when you arrive home, peckish, from a night at the theater or movies. It is astonishing how something so light and easy to prepare can be so satisfying – and filling too!)

The cooking of fish for The Obvious Diet follows the same general plan as that for chicken – the plainer the better. Grilled fish is simple, delicious, and quick to cook. All it needs is a coating of olive oil and herbs. Steamed or poached fish – either fillets or a whole fish – is wonderful too. If you like to cook fish that way, a small investment in a fish steamer is a good idea. Obviously, the traditional Hollandaise sauce usually served with steamed fish should give way to a drizzling of olive oil. If the ingredients themselves are good enough, there's no need to cover up their flavors. It's worth remembering that heavy sauces originated as a way of disguising the taste of dishes that were of dubious freshness.

Another way to prepare fish that satisfies The Obvious Diet is to cook it *en papillote,* wrapping it in aluminum foil or parchment paper with olive oil and herbs, and baking it in its own little parcel in the oven. A fine example of a dietetic recipe along these lines is the Oven-Baked Fillet of Sea Bass from *Le Dome at Home* cookbook, which you will find in Chapter Nine.

In July and August, when we do most of our cooking out of doors at our summer home in Bridgehampton, The Obvious Diet is at its easiest to achieve. In fact, if there is any single place where I came up with the bare bones of The Obvious Diet, it was here. A few years ago, I bought the most marvelous, in fact to me the best barbecue: a wood-burning contraption called The Grillery designed by a former mathematics professor at Michigan State University. The principle of the design is that the natural juices of the food you are cooking (plus, of course, the marinade) run down canted V-grooves into pans, from which you can rebaste the meat, chicken, or fish and eventually pass around at the table.

Barbecue cooking lends itself to simple recipes for fish and chicken, so here are a few of my favorites. (Certainly you can make these dishes – admittedly less successfully – using the grill of your indoor stove or a grill pan heated very hot over a burner; but even a small barbecue in your garden or terrace can produce excellent results.)

Terrifically Tasty Tuna

Marinade

¹/₄ cup soy sauce

2 garlic cloves, finely chopped

¹/₄ cup olive oil

1 tablespoon finely chopped fresh ginger (or else powdered ginger)

1 tablespoon grated orange (or lemon) zest

¹/₄ cup sherry

(*Note* These quantities can be altered easily – just make sure the olive oil, sherry, and soy sauce are combined in equal portions.)

individual tuna steaks, cut 1 to 1¹/₂ in. thick

Marinate the tuna for no less than one hour and no more than three hours (any more marinating tends to make the flesh soggy). Grill the fish according to the usual "ten minutes per inch" formula. For a steak 1 inch thick, I would grill each side for 4 minutes, hopefully achieving a burnt outside and a moist, medium rare inside. Keep basting the fish with the marinade as you cook it. Any leftover marinade can be heated and passed around with the fish.

Following is an idea for dealing with the leftovers, if any:

Ivansofe's Tuna Salad

Combine the ingredients in a bowl, add some fresh chopped parsley, a dash of extra virgin olive oil, a dash of balsamic vinegar, salt and pepper to taste.

cold, grilled tuna – enough for the number you are feeding. Or, if no leftover fresh tuna is available, use a large can of unsalted tuna, shredded.

chopped celery – one stalk per 8 oz of tuna

canned chick peas – use the same quantity of chick peas as tuna

Swordfish

As with the tuna recipe opposite, do not let the fish marinate for less than one hour or more than three hours. Grill a 1-inch-thick piece for the full ten minutes, i.e. five minutes per side, because you want to serve swordfish considerably less "rare" than tuna steaks.

Marinade

olive oil

lemon juice

lots of chopped fresh cilantro

crushed cloves of garlic

fresh ground black pepper

individual swordfish steaks, 1 in. thick

Barbecued Chicken

Marinade

equal portions of red wine and dark soy sauce

1 tablespoon olive oil per 1 cup of marinade

1 crushed clove of garlic per 1 cup of marinade

lots of freshly ground black pepper

powdered ginger (about one teaspoon)

1 chicken

The chicken should be cut into eight pieces, and marinated for about 4 hours or more (preferably in the refrigerator for the first three hours).

Make sure there is plenty of oil on the grill so that the chicken does not stick. Barbecue the chicken pieces mostly with the flesh side next to the flames. The heat should not be too intense at this point, so that the chicken cooks slowly and does not blacken on the outside while remaining raw on the inside. The skin side should cook for no more than the last five minutes of the cooking time, at which point the heat can be more intense.

Any leftover marinade can be reheated and served with the chicken as a delicious sauce.

Salmon à la Bob Cochran

A friend of mine from the Hamptons likes to fly up to Alaska each summer to fish for salmon in the St. Marguerite River. A couple of years ago, he returned with a beautiful specimen and invited a few friends over to sample his fishing triumph. His recipe was deceptively simple and fabulously tasty.

Buy a whole fillet of salmon with the skin left on, not cut into steaks.

Cover the flesh side with a mixture of olive oil and dill. Rub sea salt (or kosher salt) into the skin side after moistening with some olive oil. Let it stand for one hour.

Cook the fish by placing it on the barbecue with the skin side down. *Never turn it!* The basic principle of this recipe is that after the usual "ten minutes per inch" cooking formula has been achieved (be careful here, because the thickness of the fillet varies, especially if cut from the tail end of the fish), the skin has been seared to a delicious, crispy crust while the flesh of the salmon has been gently cooked by the indirect heat rising up from below – making it moist and tender, almost as though it had been poached rather than barbecued. Amazing! And hard to believe that something so tasty can also be good for you!

As I said above, I have tried to reduce radically – but certainly not banish totally – my intake of meat. I have also commented on how remarkably easy it was to do this after a lifetime of carnivorous eating habits. But I'm a realist too. A good grilled steak every now and then will not undo all the good you have achieved through your Obvious Dieting, and so here is a good barbecue recipe provided to me by my friend Chris Cerf:

Steak à la Chris Cerf

Marinade

equal portions of red wine, Dijon mustard, and soy sauce

very thick steaks

The secret to the success of this recipe is (a) to use a very thick steak and (b) to sear the meat for one and a half minutes on each side *before* putting on the marinade. After the first side is seared and turned, smear on the Cerf Sauce with a brush. Keep brushing on the sauce regularly, turning the meat every three minutes or so until done.

Alcohol

Alcohol is a major source of calories and one of the most frequent questions I am asked about my diet is this: can you consume alcohol on it? My answer is a barely qualified but otherwise emphatic yes. Moderate drinking, say many people who know a lot about these things, has the advantage of lowering stress levels, which is perhaps why we all know the story of leathery old French peasants who live to a hundred thanks to a glass or two of country red every day. It's achieving moderation that is the hard part for most people. I endured the total prohibition of my Obvious Diet during the first month, but I am all for moderate alcohol consumption in my long-range eating plan. Certainly it helps that, by observing your Cleansing Day, you eliminate one-seventh of your weekly alcohol intake automatically. Making it a rule never to drink alcohol at lunch also helps. You can also embark on your own personal schemes to limit (or, more accurately, moderate) your intake of alcohol. Women, who have the disadvantage of metabolizing alcohol more slowly than men, are, according to government guidelines, advised that moderation equals just one drink a day while men get away with two – I know, it's not fair!

I am all for moderate alcohol consumption in my long-range eating plan.

I believe that your diet should not be a state of siege, but a state of mind.

As I have already noted, I have, for many years, ritually given up alcohol for the month of August and occasionally for Lent as well. I can highly recommend this method of limiting your total alcohol intake. Pick a month that seems right for you (August on Long Island is hot and muggy, so it seems a good time to avoid further fumes in my brain) and just make up your mind to go without alcohol for thirty days. Another way of dealing with occasional abstinence is to take one week every month – first, last, or in-between, it really doesn't matter – and banish alcohol for those seven days. My friend Melvyn Bragg used to declare the first seven days of every month an "alcohol-free zone." Whatever permutation suits you of days/weeks/months on or off alcohol is fine. There are no hard-and-fast rules except to enjoy your tipple, but do so in moderation.

It seems to me that, although I acknowledge the drinking of alcohol puts on weight, moderate consumption does not interfere with my long-range plan to eat less, eat better, and keep myself from putting back the weight I have lost. There is a balance to be struck, and I believe alcohol can be part of that balance. Wine in particular fits the bill – a glass or two with a meal – once again taking the lead from traditional Mediterranean diets.

As you will gather from my personal plan, The Obvious Diet is not a form of torture. I believe that your diet should not be a state of siege, but a state of mind. Enjoy your food! Believe in olive oil and vinaigrette! (And, by the way, invest in the very best olive oil you can find. If olive oil starts to replace complex, intricate – and fattening – sauces in your diet, it ought to be of the highest possible quality.) Have some wine with your meal! Eat well! Live well! And still keep off the weight, just as I have done, by sticking to the few, flexible principles of The Obvious Diet.

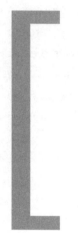

**The meat or fish
on my plate
should be no
bigger than a
deck of cards.**

Tina Brown

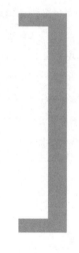

CHAPTER SIX

Living with The Obvious Diet

Several years ago, my wife and I were driving back from a fabulous lunch in a famous country restaurant with Ken and Barbara Follett. I overheard Carol say to Barbara: "Oh, I've eaten too much and have that awful overstuffed feeling!" I interjected, "I *love* that feeling!" And I meant it. I loved the feeling of heaviness, lassitude, and satiety that came with eating far too much good food. Being stuffed to the gills was then a happy state of being for me, a state I looked forward to – the sheer mindless contentment of the python who has swallowed the rabbit whole. Not any longer! Now I recognize it for what it is: an uncomfortable feeling, a sign that my system is straining to cope with excess.

The difference is that, by following the principles of The Obvious Diet, my basic assumptions about what constitutes a satisfying meal have changed. My body has become used to the far more rewarding feeling brought about by lighter eating; that old sensation of heaviness in the gut may be bearable, but it is no longer desirable. This change didn't happen overnight. It took many a tricky and challenging situation before I achieved this new, different but equally satisfying feeling: the very different feeling of the contentment that comes with eating exactly what I want to, rather than succumbing to an inner voice so loud that it drowns out all reason and the next thing I know I have eaten the greatest quantities of the heaviest foods on offer. Whereas, once upon a time in restaurants, my eyes went straight to the starred items on the menu – the *specialités de la maison,* which were invariably the heaviest dishes – I now habitually seek out the lightest dishes. It is a question of retraining your taste, and the good news is that this retraining process is easier – and far quicker – than you would ever have imagined.

In this chapter I will give you some tips on how to keep your eating within the boundaries of your Obvious Diet while living life to the full. Not only during the meals you eat at home but also your food and drink consumption at restaurants, dinner parties, cocktail receptions, hotels, and banquets (including that

You can party as much as you like (I certainly do!) and still keep the weight off.

annual ordeal of trial by food better known as Christmas). Just because you are on a constant and permanent weight control regime doesn't mean you need to stay home just munching carrot sticks in front of the TV; you can party as much as you like (I certainly do!) and still keep the weight off.

Eating at Home

Your home is the simplest place to follow your Obvious Diet, because *you* control the environment. Yes, you may have to fit your special dietary requirements into the menu planning of the other members of your family, but compared to eating out at restaurants or going to dinner parties or banquets, it is relatively easy to eat exactly the way you want.

The most important thing to remember is: Plan Ahead! Knowing well in advance what you are going to eat helps you to stay in complete control of your food and drink consumption. This is especially important if you are living with people who don't necessarily want to share your diet. You should decide no later than the night before exactly what you want to eat the next day, so the right food can be at hand for the menus you have selected. If you are the kind of person who likes to have things worked out further in advance, all well and good, go ahead and shop and plan for the whole week, but I would suggest to everybody else that the minimum is to plan for the day ahead.

It is a huge help to decide to have more or less the same breakfast every day. With the element of choice largely gone, compliance with your diet is made that much easier. Start the day right and you've set the tone for the meals to come.

Lunches and dinners at home should follow the same basic pattern: keep them simple, light, and in line with your Obvious Diet precepts. Again, I have given you some of my favorite – and most frequently eaten – recipes in the previous chapter. In a later chapter, I will provide lots of alternative recipes for these main meals of the day, but suffice it to say here that since *you* are in charge at home, there can be no excuses for straying from your healthy-eating plan. Here are a few general rules and tips for eating at home the Obvious way.

Snacks

Most people I know love to snack, which makes it vitally important to keep a supply of healthy snacks in the refrigerator for those moments when you crave a few bites of food to keep you going. I mentioned earlier my substitution of Martha Stewart's Blanched Vegetables for my pre–Obvious Diet ham chunks. These are so tasty that they also make a perfect healthy snack for the sweet-toothed dieter. Opposite is the recipe:

Vegetables in Mustard Vinaigrette

Serves 20

1 head of cauliflower, cut into florets

1 head of broccoli, cut into florets

1 lb asparagus, trimmed

1 lb string beans

6 oz sugar snaps or snow peas

1 lb carrots, peeled with a little of the tops intact

Mustard Vinaigrette

3 oz tarragon vinegar or Japanese rice vinegar

2 tablespoons Dijon mustard

1 cup olive oil (for a lighter dressing, use half vegetable oil)

coarse kosher or sea salt to taste

freshly ground black pepper

1 shallot, finely minced

chopped fresh tarragon, chervil, dill, and flat-leaf parsley (optional)

In separate pots of boiling, lightly salted water, blanch the vegetables until just tender. Drain, refresh in ice water, and drain again. Dry the vegetables well and arrange decoratively on a platter.

To make the mustard vinaigrette, whisk the vinegar and mustard together. Add the oil a few drops at a time, whisking vigorously. Season with salt, pepper, shallot, and herbs. Whisk again before spooning over vegetables.

Vinaigrette may be made in advance. Store in the refrigerator, but do not add the shallot and herbs until ready to use. If it solidifies, let it stand at room temperature until it can be whisked into a creamy dressing.

(*Note* The quantities are large – 20 servings – because this dish is intended to be passed around at parties. Either make lots of it to keep in the fridge for snacking, or the quantities can be easily adjusted downward.)

In addition to your supply of dietetic snacks (be they raw or cooked vegetables, fresh fruit, olives, hard-boiled eggs, etc.) always keep some vegetable soup, consommé, or clear broth in the fridge. It not only makes a good liquid snack, if you are so inclined, but a bowl of soup at lunch or dinner can fill you up in a healthy and dietetic manner so that you end up eating less over the course of the day. In my own case, I always keep a supply of my Cleansing Day Cabbage Soup in the freezer, so I can use it for regular mealtimes during the week. And if, for example, you feel you have had too much for lunch – or your dinner is for some reason delayed until late in the evening – it makes a perfect light meal on its own or with some mixed salad on the side.

Fruit

Always have a fabulous selection of fruits available. You will be surprised at how many exotic fruits you will find on sale in most greengrocers and supermarkets these days. Papayas, mangoes, melons, pomegranates ... the list of delicious fruits goes on and on.

One fruit that always satisfies the Obvious Dieter is the humble banana. It is wonderfully portable, and makes a great snack on the move – especially in

One fruit that always satisfies the Obvious Dieter is the humble banana.

the car. (But don't let the police see you eating it!) Finally, apart from their value to you as dietetic snacks, displays of fresh fruit are aesthetically very pleasing too!

Herbs and Spices

Herbs and spices take on a new importance for the Obvious Dieter at home. If you are trying to keep your meals as simple and healthy as possible – chicken, fish, and lean meat rather than stews and roasts, grilled or poached food rather than fried, simple vegetables rather than concoctions drowning in creamy sauces, less rather than more – your taste buds will benefit from imaginative use of herbs and spices. Experiment! Try grilled chicken or fish with a variety of different herbs. Try new and different spices to make variations on some of your favorite dishes. As I have said, The Obvious Diet should not be a form of torture.

Smaller Servings

Just as I advise you always to leave some food on your plate at restaurants, try to limit your intake at home as well by serving smaller portions. Family-style meals work well, because you can take what you want – small amounts – from the serving bowls as they make their rounds.

The Sweet Tooth

If you find you can keep to your rules for the main course, but then crave something sweet to finish off (and fruit just won't do it), try one small piece of the best-quality chocolate you can afford. Better this than succumbing to a cheap, fat-laden chocolate bar or tub of ice cream.

Brush Your Teeth!

Another useful hint for curbing your appetite when dining at home is to make a detour to the bathroom to brush your teeth on your way to the dining room! When you arrive at the dinner table with a freshly cleaned mouth, you are somehow less likely to stuff yourself. Try it!

Eating at Restaurants

One night several years ago my wife and I arrived at the Ivy Restaurant around 9:30 p.m. for dinner. When Mitchell Everard, the headwaiter, came to the table to take our order, I said, "Mitchell, all I feel like eating tonight is a big bowl of salad, with everything the chef wants to throw into it." A confession is in order at this point: since this scene took place in my pre–Obvious Diet days, I also ordered a plate of the Ivy's fabulous *pommes allumettes* with mayonnaise instead of ketchup! Then, as I looked around the restaurant and saw how busy it was, I felt guilty about putting in a special order when the place was so packed. People were flooding in – Tony Blair (then the Leader of the Opposition) arrived with a party of friends; John Cleese came in just after him – and waiters were scurrying around tables of the great and good of London, all clamoring for their meals. So, I called Mitchell over and asked him not to bother about my special order and bring me back the menu so I could just order a normal dish. "Nonsense, Ed!" he said. "You have no idea what a pleasure it is to have a customer feel relaxed enough to ask the kitchen for whatever he wants. It means we're doing our job properly."

Contrast this attitude with a recent experience I had at some new and rather pretentious eatery in St. John's Wood. The menu was one of those fashionable "fusion" efforts – Italian, Californian, Moroccan, you-name-it we-complicate-it jumble food – and everything on the menu seemed to contain things (goat cheese, croutons, etc.) that were not on my Obvious Diet. I asked the waitress if the chef could make me a simple mixed or green salad with a vinaigrette dressing. "I'm afraid our chef doesn't allow any changes or substitutions on the menu, sir," she announced grandly. And I knew right then that this was the last time I'd ever set foot in the place.

> **The jumped-up local says "absolutely not," yet one of the most famous and prestigious restaurants in the world says "yes."**

The jumped-up local says "absolutely not," yet one of the most famous and prestigious restaurants in the world says "yes."

The restaurant with a waiting list lasting weeks is accommodating; the one with a reputation to make won't deviate from its foodie pretensions.

Any restaurant worth its salt should, at your request, be able to make you a simple alternative to the dishes on their menu. It figures, when you think about it: the better the restaurant, the more skillful they are at satisfying their customers! I recall eating at one of the most elegant restaurants in New York City – the Grill Room at the Four Seasons – with my friend Michael Korda, the famous publisher and author. He always ordered exactly the same meal, which was certainly not on the menu but quite probably on his own personal Obvious Diet: a baked potato with a chopped salad on the side. No one ever blinked an eye at his choice; they were just delighted to bring it to him.

You should never be afraid to order *exactly* what you want in restaurants.

If there are no starters that make diet sense to you, then ask for a salad. If there is a starter that you want as a main course – either in a starter portion or larger – then just ask for

You should never be afraid to order *exactly* what you want in restaurants.

it. If a dish you desire comes with sauce, ask for it to be served on the side – so that *you* (and not some sous-chef in the kitchen) decide how much of it you want to have on your food. Usually, most chicken, fish, or meat dishes found on the menu can be served plainly grilled, if requested. Ingredients can be dropped ("No potatoes with that, please") or added ("Please add some sliced tomatoes to the arugula salad"). Just ask! Restaurants exist to cater to their customers – that's why you go there in the first place.

Although you can, to a certain extent, control *what* you eat in a restaurant, you cannot control *how much* food they will put on your plate. If it's more than you want, either leave some, or else ask for a doggy-bag; you paid for it, so why not take it home and eat it there the next day?

Never eat a three-course meal.

Never eat a three-course meal. Order two appetizers, or even just one main course. If you must have dessert, skip another course, as three is just too much food!

If you are going to try a very special restaurant – one of those multi-starred Michelin "temples of gastronomy" where we occasionally need to worship – I suggest you save up the experience for your Treat Meal of the week. Then you can order their signature dishes with impunity and without guilt (although I can confidently predict, you will feel less and less like consuming heavy food once you are well embarked on your Obvious Diet).

On the Move

Traveling presents its own problems to the Obvious Dieter. First of all, eating on airplanes – no matter what class you fly – is certainly not going to be a memorable culinary experience, to say the very least. I sometimes think that the only reason they serve food on airplanes is to make sure that most of the passengers are seated most of the time, rather than clogging up the aisles. Obviously speaking, the best approach to eating on a plane is not to eat at all. However, if you are really very hungry, you may find that your dreary little plastic tray has some salad or fruit on it: eat that, not the main course, unless it has some edible vegetables. Never eat fish – cooked or smoked – on a plane. If anything is going to go wrong with airplane food, fish is the prime candidate for giving you food poisoning. If you can remember to arrange it before you fly, you are probably best off ordering a vegetarian meal – but there is no guarantee of that, because even

The only truly memorable meal I ever had in a lifetime of air travel was on the Concorde.

vegetarian meals can be pretty stodgy and awful!

The only truly memorable meal I ever had in a lifetime of air travel was on the Concorde, where I was once served a plate of excellent cold grouse and salad, with some superb claret. But that meal was one out of (literally) thousands – and, given the cost of flying the Concorde in those days, actually cost me thousands!

Wherever you are, the same rules apply – order the plainest dishes, sauce on the side.

Otherwise, the best strategy is to stay hungry until you arrive at your destination. Or do what I sometimes do if I have a few minutes to spare before boarding. Go and buy some delicious treat at one of the more luxurious airport shops – some caviar or smoked salmon, for example – and then ask the stewardess to serve it to you on a plate. They never refuse if asked nicely. Another frequent traveler's tip, for those interested in minimizing the ill-effects of hours in the air, is to avoid or minimize alcohol, as it further dehydrates what, after a flight, is your already dehydrated body.

When you are on the road, you not only have to cope with strange hotels and restaurants where you don't know the ropes, but you might find yourself wrestling with menus in a foreign language. Nevertheless, wherever you are, the same rules apply. Order the plainest dishes, sauce on the side. *Always ask for what you want!* You're not going to win friends and influence people by stoically swallowing heavy stodge when you only wanted a light snack.

If you are ordering from room service in hotels, stick to the salads – forget about club sandwiches oozing mayonnaise or cheeseburgers with fries. In foreign restaurants, drop or add ingredients as you wish, just as you would at home. A phrase-book might assist you here, or a pointing finger – if you see something you'd like to eat at another table, point it out to the waiter who is asking for your order – the food isn't going to take offense. As ever, eat only two courses. If you know of a restaurant specializing in fish rather than meat, choose it; it's always less fattening! It's hard, of course, to resist the local goodies – especially if, like me, you are a frequent traveler to France or Italy. But because the ingredients are so good in those countries, even the plainest food still dazzles. As they say, the mark of a really great chef is how well he does the simple things. What's more, now that you are treating your body as it should be treated, those *grandes bouffes* of old won't be all that appealing anyway. Especially if you remember how you used to feel afterward. I remember once lying miserably in a hotel bedroom in Paris after consuming an ingot of the greatest *foie gras* in France at that divine little hole-in-the-wall restaurant L'Ami Louis – more or less praying for death because I felt as stuffed as the poor goose had been!

Banquets

All of us have suffered at one time or another through the mediocre catered food at weddings, charity galas, anniversary dinners, club nights, etc. One of the occupational hazards of the publishing business is the number of celebratory dinners at long tables where someone else – looking for the lowest common denominator which will successfully engage the taste buds of all and sundry – has chosen the food for dozens, if not hundreds, of people. Here's how to cope.

If you know in advance what's on the eating agenda, you can act accordingly.

Try to find out the menu *before* you arrive. If that's impossible, then check it out as soon as you get to the venue.

If you know in advance what's on the eating agenda, you can act accordingly: pass up courses without worrying that you'll go hungry if you know there's something you can/you'd like to eat coming later, or fill up on an early course that appeals, and then use your mouth for talking, not eating.

Even better, as unobtrusively as you can manage, find the headwaiter and ask for the vegetarian alternative, which is usually available at such functions. I recently attended the annual Fulbright Commission dinner at a large London hotel and saw that the menu was full of things that were off my Obvious Diet. I whispered in the ear of the headwaiter, and, while everyone at the table was served a tired-looking starter of Parma ham and soggy melon, I was enjoying some plump, delicious asparagus with a passable vinaigrette sauce. Many jealous eyes fell on my plate! And while my table mates were grimly sawing their way through some tough tournedos, I had a perfectly acceptable piece of grilled salmon for my main course. At the end of the meal, when some hideously fattening dessert is invariably brought in, you can always order a fruit plate – as long as you're not following the food combining "no fruit after meals" approach as part of your Obvious Diet.

Cocktail Parties

As the old saying goes, "If I had a dollar for every cocktail party I've attended in my forty-plus years in publishing ..."

The cocktail party is dangerous ground for the Obvious Dieter. Waiters pour very aggressively, so you could end up imbibing more than the "moderate" amount of alcohol you may have allowed yourself on your diet. If you can bear it, just drink water or juice – it's always an amusing experience to hear the volume

The cocktail party is dangerous ground for the Obvious Dieter.

go up and the quality of the conversation go down in a room full of drinkers while you remain sober! To keep a firm grip on how much alcohol you are downing, don't be afraid to put your hand over the top of your glass – there will always be another waiter along in a minute. Otherwise, make it a point to drink alternate glasses of wine and water. Or order a "spritzer" – half a glass of white wine, topped up with sparkling water – a refreshing, but not at all lethal, tipple.

Canapés are also served aggressively, and you must be careful about consuming too many of them because they are often very fattening concoctions. My strategy is to eat only those canapés from which I can remove the treat from its base. To do this, you must clearly be willing to use your fingers and endure the stares of those who find this activity rather unsavory. I recently attended a cocktail party at the extremely grand British Embassy Residence in Paris to celebrate the French publication of my client Frederick Forsyth's latest book. The wife of the British ambassador, Lady Jay, has made a great effort to provide delicious (and quintessentially British) snacks at the Embassy parties. Wanting to sample these goodies – but not the bread or pastry on which they were served – I went through my customary ritual of separating the two with my fingers. The bases went into the ashtrays, the treat into my mouth, any residue on my finger onto the cocktail napkin. Every now and then, a liveried member of staff, with great aplomb, would remove the bread from the ashtray in exactly the same way he would have dealt with a cigarette butt, a look of detached tolerance on his face. No one batted an eyelash at my anti-wheat/yeast/gluten tactics.

The point here is, once again, you must not be afraid to ask for the things you want, to decline or remove the things you don't want, to do the things you need to do to follow your Obvious Diet. Just as you are the person who best knows your eating habits, likes, dislikes, and needs, you are the person you have to rely on to put what you know about yourself into effect.

You make the rules, and you police them: that's the deal. Nowhere is it written in the game plan – or in any guides to etiquette as far as I know – that you are condemned to eat and drink what everyone else in the room is eating and drinking. You have a choice and you should not be afraid or embarrassed to exercise it! (A delightful postscript: several months after the party, I bumped into Lady Jay at the opening night of the Chelsea Flower Show and confessed what I had done with her canapés. She totally approved!)

You make the rules, and you police them: that's the deal.

Dinner Parties

Your ability to follow The Obvious Diet while dining at the homes of your friends is in direct proportion to how close the friends are to you. Really close friends are those you can ask to tailor the meal – or, at the very least, *your* part of the meal – to your dieting needs. The easiest invitations of all come with a polite inquiry whether there are any foods you don't eat or habitually avoid. If this is not a customary practice in your circle of friends, then you can make it one next time you invite people over for a meal.

> **Take a few face-saving bites and then spread the rest artfully around the plate.**

When all else fails, you should be able to rely on a good friend either making you an omelette or serving you a plate of smoked salmon, if the meal they are serving that night is too rich for your diet. If, however, you are dining with people you don't know very well, then manipulation of the menu is often not possible and you must deal with the meal as and when it comes. My basic approach in this case is to do what kids do, namely, to take a few face-saving bites and then spread the rest artfully around the plate.

At our home, my wife and I tend to cater for possible dieters among our invitees by serving meals that are simple and not overly rich. Incidentally, we did this long before I fell under the spell of The Obvious Diet, because it seemed to us a considerate thing to do. So, at our table, there are always plenty of salads and vegetables, and the main course is, more often than not, plainly roasted organic chicken.

"Keep it simple" is great advice for giving dinner to friends. And no one does it better than our friends Ruth and Richard Rogers. If anyone could prepare and serve a fancy, restaurant-style meal at home, it is Ruth Rogers, co-owner with Rose Gray of the justly famous River Cafe. But dinner at their gorgeous Chelsea home is *always* simple and *always* a pleasure. While chatting with you over a glass of wine and some olives in her kitchen, Ruth will invariably be preparing some delicious salads and vegetables, and then simply grilling some fresh fish with herbs. Last time we dined there, we had superb wild salmon served with a spicy chili sauce, cannellini beans, oven-roasted tomatoes with garlic, and a plain arugula salad. Dessert was cheese followed by raspberries. Nothing could have been simpler or tastier.

"Keep it simple" is great advice for giving dinner to friends.

Once again, the message is that living with The Obvious Diet on the road or at parties and restaurants is, like so many other things in life, a question of balance. You must balance your determination to eat simply and dietetically with the demands of your social and professional life. Try to adapt your eating to the situation in which you find yourself and do the best you can without upsetting too many people – most especially yourself! If you know that it will be difficult to avoid eating too much forbidden food at an upcoming social occasion, then make sure you eat very lightly during the other meals of the day – the meals over which you *are* in control. Alternatively, go easy on what's put in front of you and fill up on something tasty and healthy at home later. It is, after all, the totality of your food intake that you need to worry about, not one rogue meal! Remember that The Obvious Diet is not an exact science, but an overarching commitment to eating less and eating better. You should never be trapped in commitments that are impossible to keep, or the only thing you are certain to achieve is failure. Keep to the commitments that are possible and you can live the kind of life you want to live – but still keep your weight under control.

Christmas

Christmas comes but once a year, which is a relief to the millions of people who, by December 27, have eaten themselves into a stupor and collapsed in front of the television to watch the inevitable action movie, and who, when the final explosions fill the screen, suspect that they too are on the verge of blowing up. Familiar with the feeling? Who isn't? And who hasn't made a New Year's resolution there and then to go on a diet and to never, ever, sink to such extreme gluttony again.

The obvious thing about Christmas is that there's going to be a lot of food around.

The obvious thing about Christmas is that there's going to be a lot of food around. And then a lot of leftover food clogging up the fridge until you and your next of kin have eaten your way through it all. Equally obvious is that it's hard to resist such tasty fare or to turn down dish after dish prepared by a family member without offending. Which brings us to the obvious tactic for Christmas: the easiest way to deal with Christmas on The Obvious Diet is to declare the day your Treat Meal (more in the next chapter), do your worst (or best), and then return to the usual regime. If you've already tasted the good stuff on the day itself, it should be no great sacrifice to stay away from the much diminished two-day-old leftovers.

If you are feeling particularly saintly, of course, you can adopt other stratagems and stick as close as you can to your normal regime. When you go to all those parties leading up to Christmas, just follow the rules I gave you in the Cocktail

Parties section of this chapter. And, on The Day itself, try to avoid the turkey skin and the stuffing, turn up your nose at the Christmas cake and hard sauce, and don't go in for a second – well, it's Christmas, you can allow yourself a little celebration – let's say third helping.

If you eat mainly vegetables and fruit on your diet, not only will you lose weight, but it will also help to detox your body.

Marie Helvin

CHAPTER SEVEN

The Cleansing Day/Treat Meal

A diet book is not the place people go to find eternal truths about humanity. You don't need me to tell you that every one of us has a good and a bad side. It's common knowledge that we all encompass aspects of saint and sinner, an angel in white on one shoulder whispering in our ear to be good and virtuous and stick to the straight and narrow, and, in opposition, a little pointy-tailed red guy prodding us with his fork, trying to get us to abandon our good intentions and fall back into our old ways.

The Obvious Diet acknowledges these two warring sides of our human nature in its two weekly rituals: the Cleansing Day and the Treat Meal. One procedure involves a certain amount of abstention, a day of sustenance involving a reduced intake of food, but very healthy food at that! The Treat Meal recognises that there are certain meals, certain foods that nobody could ever contemplate banishing from their lives forever — favorite dishes which, no matter how calorific or fattening, are just "too good to resist." The Obvious Diet takes account of these cravings and, instead of taking the totally unrealistic position that they will be prohibited "forever," allows you 52 meals of your absolute choice every year – quite a bit of sinfulness for any sinner, but not enough to knock you off your generally saintly course in any significant way.

The Cleansing Day

It is obvious that six rather than seven days of eating can make a substantial contribution to keeping your weight under control. But there's more to it than that. A day off food, or in the case of The Obvious Diet, a day when all you eat is healthful fruit and vegetables, gives the system a rest, and helps the body eliminate toxins and rejuvenate.

The seed for this tenet of The Obvious Diet plan, and for a relatively protein-free day as part of my life, came from my friend and client Dr. Ali, who incorporated it into the treatment notes he wrote for me after our first consultation.

Fasting is so natural that it has been codified into practically every major world religion. I continue to be fascinated by the response from people I tell about my Cleansing Day, how many of them have parents or grandparents who

Fasting is so natural that it has been codified into practically every major world religion.

swore by a regimen of one day off food every week.

It's obvious that a total fast will result in rapid weight loss; no calories going in forces the body to seek alternate sources of energy, starting with the fat it has stored up for just such an eventuality. It's equally obvious, as any regular dieter knows through bitter personal experience, that as soon as you start to eat regularly again, the body will try and store up every calorie it can as fat in preparation for what it fears is the next famine, with the all too predictable result that your weight is likely to increase rather than decrease over the long term.

But my Cleansing Day is not a fast *per se*, since you can drink unlimited juice and eat as much as you want as long as it's fruit, raw vegetables, salad, and vegetable soup. It is also very important that you drink lots of water on the Cleansing Day – at least 6 to 8 glasses per day, and even more if you want. Drinking water is a good idea anyway, since often a glass of water is really what the body wants when we feel a pang of appetite. But you should stick to still water – not the sparkling variety, which tends to give you a bloated feeling (if not figure). Or get inventive – even plain water can be jazzed up:

Combine, in a pitcher:
Good bottled or filtered water (still, not sparkling)
A few slices of lemon, orange, and cucumber
Place in fridge until cold.

Of course, if you feel that you want to incorporate a full-blown fast in your own Obvious Diet, then I suggest you follow the precepts my client Marie Helvin laid out in her excellent book on the subject, *Bodypure*.

Daunting as it may sound, the Cleansing Day is much easier to get through than you would imagine. It's not a question of exalted spiritual achievement, but the replacement of your standard three meals a day with lighter, healthier alternatives for one day a week. And the great reward is that the next day you will feel lighter and full of energy – I guarantee! And, who knows, you may even experience that rare feeling of genuine hunger, the body sending out the impulse to eat not out of habit, not to seek comfort, not to find solace, not because other people are eating, but because your body clearly, naturally, wants fuel and sustenance.

I believe it is important that you choose a regular day of the week for your Cleansing Day.

I have picked Sunday because it is a day that, for me, is usually free of any significant social or business obligations and commitments – and free of the eating implications that frequently accompany those occasions. As often

It is important that you choose a regular day of the week for your Cleansing Day.

as I can, I try to play golf at my club on Sundays, so that when lunchtime comes around I am usually outdoors, pulling my cart around the course and enjoying the fresh air and the golf. By the time I get home in the late afternoon, a few pieces of fruit or crudités can allay any afternoon hunger pangs, and then supper can be simply some vegetable soup or salad – or a bit of both. Although I like the regularity of my Sunday Cleansing Days, I sometimes vary which day of the week it is to fit in with my schedule. Of course, the day you pick should be the one that's going to be easiest for you to stick to.

The Cleansing Day is one of the few hard-and-fast rules in the whole Obvious Diet, so you must try to make available at least one day a week for this ritual as a vital contribution to your continued weight control plan! Another good candidate for your Cleansing Day is a day which you spend traveling. I go back and forth to the U.S. very often, and long hours on an airplane provide an ideal context in which to eat only fruit or salad – and a bonus is that eating light is a good way to minimize any jet lag problems.

I consciously try to drink a lot of fluids during this Cleansing Day, in accordance with Dr. Ali's general nutritional advice. I keep a big supply of my two favorite juices – cranberry juice and V8 juice – in the kitchen cupboard, and help myself to them as often as I can. Another good idea is to leave bottles of water – I prefer still water (e.g., Evian) to sparkling water, as I don't want to imbibe all that bloating gas

– all over the house, so that I can have a few sips wherever I happen to be, whenever I want, and nip any superfluous hunger pangs in the bud.

As I have already mentioned, the soup I use as the basis for my Cleansing Day is the Cabbage Soup from the Sacred Heart Memorial Hospital 7 Day Fat Burning Diet (aka The Cabbage Soup Diet). Here is the recipe:

Cabbage Soup

Chop vegetables, put together with tomatoes and stock cubes in a saucepan, cover with water and bring to the boil. Cover and simmer until all the vegetables are tender.

This soup can be eaten anytime you are hungry. Eat as much as you want, whenever you want, throughout the day.

2 large onions

2 green peppers

1 large cabbage

1 bunch of celery

2 cans tomatoes

2 stock cubes

salt and pepper

parsley

herbs (or hot sauce or curry powder) as desired

If this particular vegetable soup doesn't appeal to you, then I can offer two more vegetable soup recipes from my client Nigella Lawson's already classic *How to Eat* that are equally appropriate – and perhaps more to your taste!

Vegetable Miso Broth

This is essential to my low-fat eating moments. I cook it more frequently than I cook anything else, and every time I do I make it differently. Basically, I just boil, in salted water, various vegetables, any that I feel like, putting them in the pan in the order they'll take to cook (thus turnips first, watercress last) and then drain them into a bowl. Into this bowl I pour a pitcher of salty soup made out of some vegetable bouillon powder and 1 tablespoon of miso. Sometimes I add ginger to the broth and stir in some pickled ginger while I'm eating it. But mostly it's just plain vegetables, chunked and still crunchy, with that almost creatively, emphatically aromatic, miso-thickened broth.

The quantities I give on the following page are to be viewed as sketchy; ignore or add to them as you wish.

Put a large pan of water on to boil and when boiling add salt. Then add the turnips. After about 5 minutes, add the carrots. After another 7 or so minutes, add the broccoli. Give this 2 to 3 minutes, then chuck in the zucchini, and after another minute the sugar snap peas. Just as you're about to drain the pan, throw in the watercress and then empty the entire contents into a colander in the sink.

Meanwhile make the broth. Pour 2 cups boiling water from the kettle into a pitcher and stir in 2 teaspoons vegetable bouillon, and then 1 heaping teaspoon (or more to taste) miso. Put the drained vegetables into a pasta bowl, then pour over the miso broth. Add chopped parsley or cilantro if wished. Eat.

Serves 4

2 turnips, peeled and quartered

1 carrot, peeled and cut into large, chunky sticks

a few florets broccoli

1 zucchini, halved lengthwise and then halved across

handful of sugar snap peas, each chopped into 2–3 pieces

handful watercress

2 teaspoons vegetable bouillon powder

1 heaping teaspoon miso powder

fresh parsley or cilantro, chopped (optional)

Vegetable Soup

A vegetable soup doesn't require a recipe, and I certainly don't want to suggest you get out your scales to make it with mechanical accuracy. But it's helpful to have a working model for a plain but infinitely variable soup. This one is not exactly the mix of carrot, parsnip, and turnip my mother used to make, and which we knew as nip soup, but is based on its memory.

I use my beloved vegetable bouillon powder most of the time, but if I've got some good organic vegetables that taste properly and vigorously of themselves, I use water. A friend of mine swears that if you use Evian or other bottled still water it makes all the difference, but I haven't quite got around to that yet.

Although my hand is pretty well (permanently) stuck, culinarily speaking, around the neck of a bottle of Marsala, I admit that there isn't a vegetable soup in the land that doesn't benefit from the addition of a little dry sherry.

Peel and roughly chop the carrots, onion, turnip, parsnip, and potato. Chop the celery and thickly slice the leek. Put the whole lot in the processor and blitz it briefly until chopped medium-fine. Obviously you needn't use the machine; I've just got into this lazy habit.

Heat the oil or butter with its drop of oil in a large wide pan (one which has a lid, preferably) and then add the chopped vegetables to it, turning them over a few times so they all have a slight slick of fat. Sprinkle with salt, cover, and on a low heat, let them half-fry, half-braise until softened, about 10 to 15 minutes, shaking the pan from time to time and occasionally opening the lid to stir (making sure nothing's sticking or burning at the bottom) before putting the lid back on again. Pour in the stock, adding the *bouquet garni* and a good grind of pepper, bring, uncovered, to a simmer, then cook for about 20 to 40 minutes (exactly how long depends on the age of the vegetables, the size you've chopped them, the dimensions of the pan,

Serves 4

2 carrots

1 onion

1 turnip

1 parsnip

1 potato

1 stalk celery

1 leek, white part only

3 tablespoons olive oil, or 1 tablespoon butter and a drop of oil

salt and pepper

7 cups vegetable stock

1 *bouquet garni*

nutmeg

1–2 tablespoons dry sherry

fresh parsley, chives, or chervil to sprinkle over when eating

and the material of which the pan's made).

When the soup's cooked, blend or process it, or push it through a food mill. Alternatively, if you've got one of those hand blenders, you can do an agreeably rough purée in the pot. Sometimes, I take out a couple of ladlefuls, blend or process them, and put them back into the soup to thicken it, without turning it all to mush. Season to taste (I like a bit of grated nutmeg at the end) and stir in the sherry before serving, sprinkling over fresh herbs as you wish.

If none of these recipes appeals, by all means substitute your own favorite vegetable soup – but please make sure that there is absolutely no butter or cream involved in the prep-aration, or you will compromise the basic premise of the Cleansing Day!

As for the salad part of your Cleansing Day, I leave this entirely to you and your sense of giving your body (and espe-cially your digestive system) a day off. Certainly you will serve the purpose of the day better by avoiding vinaigrette dressing or olive oil and sticking to plain, raw vegetables. I tend to eat the Martha Stewart vegetables, minus the delicious vinaigrette sauce, on my Cleansing Days, but the bottom line is do what you have to do. Fruit is, of course, always fruit – delicious and dietetic. I strongly recommend that you keep a good supply of your favorite fruit on hand to eat during these days.

The Treat Meal

The flip side of the Cleansing Day coin is the Treat Meal. Once a week, The Obvious Diet entitles you to a meal of your choice. That's right: absolutely *whatever* you want to eat! Let's face it – most of us, most of the time, cave in to our appetites; we tend to be greedy eaters, and each of us has our own specific foods which trigger ultimate eating satisfaction. In my case, as I have confessed, my personal weakness is for animal fat. It may, in your case, be desserts or chocolate. A diet that tries to banish certain cherished foods from your life forever is a diet that begs to be disobeyed – and eventually be abandoned altogether. It's natural for you to crave certain foods, certain meals – just as it's natural for you to want to keep your weight

A diet that tries to banish certain cherished foods from your life forever is a diet that begs to be disobeyed.

under control. The two *can* go together: if you limit your consumption of those foods to one time per week – that is fifty-two times per year – there's no serious harm to the long-term weight control program you have embarked upon, and no excuse for plunging headlong into the wrong kind of eating for the rest of the week. If anything, having that one wicked meal per week will help ensure that you stick more than ever to your overall game plan because you are actually allowed to consume your forbidden fruit on a fairly regular basis.

When I daydream about food, it is always about fatty foods: a giant corned beef or pastrami sandwich on rye bread (with coleslaw, fries, and a can of Dr. Brown's cream soda) at Katz's Deli on Houston Street in New York, the divine potato pie which accompanies the best roast chicken in the world at L'Ami Louis in Paris, the Cobb salad followed by braised short ribs of beef (with O'Brien potatoes) at The Grill in Beverly Hills, the giant sirloin steak at Peter Luger's Steakhouse in Brooklyn, New York, the equally gigantic grilled veal chop at Elaine's Restaurant in New York, a large bacon–blue cheese burger with fries at any Hamburger Hamlet branch in Los Angeles, the *filets de harengs pommes à l'huile* followed by the *pied de porc* or the *boeuf gros sel* at the Brasserie Lipp in Paris…. I could go on and on about my favorite meals, as I'm sure you could about yours – things you love to cook and eat at home, special favorite meals or desserts at particularly favorite restaurants, memorable occasions you would love to revisit, given half the chance. The advantage of The Obvious Diet is that your reward for sticking to the program week after week is that you are allowed to indulge in your favorite food fantasies – even if it is just once a week instead of all week long.

As an example of a Treat Meal, and for your amusement, I will give you the recipe for one of my favorite, fattening comfort food meals – meatloaf with kasha – followed by a contrasting, alternative version from my son Ivan and daughter-in-law Sophie (healthy L.A. people!) that follows the generally low-fat principles of The Obvious Diet:

My Meatloaf with Kasha

Preheat the oven to 350°F.

Finely dice the onion and fry it in the chicken fat until it is golden brown. Stir the chicken fat and onion mixture into the ground beef. Add the beaten egg to the mixture. Then stir in enough bread-crumbs to give the beef a nice, firm texture. Use your hands to knead every-thing! Then shape the beef mixture into a loaf, put it in a loaf pan and cover it completely with strips of bacon. Bake for one hour.

1 large onion

generous amount of chicken fat (if unavailable use mixture of butter and olive oil)

2 lb ground beef

1 beaten egg

white breadcrumbs

bacon

Kasha

1 cup buckwheat groats
1 beaten egg
salt to taste

Put one cup buckwheat groats in the bottom of a pan with one beaten egg. Stir madly over very high heat until all the grains have separated. When all the grains have been coated with the egg, add 1 cup boiling water (NOT cold water!) and salt to taste and stir. Immediately cover the pan, lower the heat and simmer for twenty minutes.

When the meatloaf has cooked, there will be plenty of juices (well, yes, fatty juices) in the roasting pan which can be used to moisten the kasha. The whole thing is insanely good to my taste buds – and very bad for me!

On the following page is a dietetic version of the same dish.

Ivansofe's Turkey Meatloaf

Preheat the oven to 400°F.

Mix all ingredients, pack the mixture into a loaf pan greased with olive oil and bake in oven for fifty minutes or so.

2 lb lean ground turkey

3 oz (or so) raw oats

$^1/_2$ chopped onion

two chopped cloves of garlic

splash of olive oil

1 large sun-dried tomato, cut up

salt and pepper to taste

herb of choice – parsley, oregano

1 egg (optional) – if not, use more olive oil

chili pepper flakes (optional)

Taste tests aside – I am salivating at the thought – the most important thing I can tell you about the Treat Meal from my own experience is that, after several weeks or months on The Obvious Diet, a strange thing will start happening to you: you will not want the same kinds of Treat Meals as you thought – the heavy, fat- or sugar-laden dishes that in the past have proven to be your downfall. What's more, even if you do consume them, you will not eat as much as you used to, nor will you feel the same contentment afterwards. And if you do, well, that's what the Treat Meal is there for, a reward and an outlet for cravings that would otherwise be difficult to control.

The Obvious Diet, as I have said, is a retraining of your eating habits and your appetites; after a few weeks, chances are you will take pleasure in the feeling of lightness after eating, rather than heaviness after the abandon of indulgence, and so this kind of eating becomes somewhat alien to you. It's not that you no longer enjoy these familiar but now exotic foods – you certainly do – but you don't want to eat as much of them – or eat them as often – as you used to.

There you have it: the Cleansing Day and the Treat Meal provide the punctuation marks to a typical week on The Obvious Diet. Stick to the principles of the diet you have designed for yourself during the week, religiously observe the Cleansing Day, treat yourself to whatever you want to have once every seven days, and you are all set to achieve the goal of keeping off the weight you lost in your first month forever and succeed where in the past you may have failed.

The Cleansing Day and the Treat Meal provide the punctuation marks.

Before attending cocktail parties, I stuff my pockets with slices of radish, cucumber, and baby carrots to nibble on.

Art Cooper

CHAPTER EIGHT

How They Do It:

The Secrets of Famous People

Have you ever noticed how often the conversation over a meal turns to the subject of eating? And have you also noticed how often that conversation focuses specifically on dieting? We seem to be equally obsessed by eating on the one hand, and by keeping our weight off (despite our eating!) on the other. Everybody I know has his own favorite method of dieting, and I'm sure your experience with your own friends is the same. When I decided to write this book, I asked my friends to help me by contributing their own diet tips and special dietetic recipes. Not surprisingly, given our universal obsession with food and diets, many of them were eager to share their dieting secrets with you.

In the following pages you'll find other people's specific tips and tricks, and the reassuring knowledge that pretty much all of us are in the same boat when it comes to food and weight and how we feel about ourselves and how much we all have to strive to keep things under control.

So come and sit around this virtual table and see what people have to say. I'm sure you will find it interesting; I certainly did!

Nan Kempner

Nan Kempner's reputation as a goddess of fashion means she is more famous than anyone I know for being perfectly thin. No wonder she is able to wear all those couture dresses so beautifully. As with everyone else, she chooses what she eats very carefully, and her suggestion about lettuce sandwiches must be one of the most original diet tips I ever heard!

When thinking about people who are overweight, you should also think about people who are underweight and have to put weight on. The same principle applies to both sets of people. To lose weight eat small amounts less often, to gain weight, eat small amounts more often. You should not deprive yourself.

Eat little of what you enjoy, that way you will not be craving all the things which are missing. Convince yourself that you are not hungry and you won't be. Do not eat everything on your plate. Having said that, cut out bread and potatoes and fattening foods. Have self-control and exercise regularly.

Watch the weight come off slowly. Judge weight loss by looking in the mirror, particularly a back view. Also judge by the fit of your clothes. Remember, moderation.

A Particular Diet Recipe:

Cut two very thick pieces of lettuce and fill them with almost anything you like, e.g., tuna and mayonnaise, cheese, or eggs and eat twice a day. These lettuce sandwiches are filling and satisfying.

Always have a drink in the evening.

Watch out that you don't get too thin.

Anne Robinson

Annie is my friend and client, and a woman I admire passionately for her style, her energy, her talent, her discipline. She is as steely about her eating as she is about every task she undertakes – as you will see from her notes about how she keeps her weight under control.

I'm sick of being told what makes me fat. I long for someone to help me stop eating. I want to know how not to run to the fridge every time I feel angry, lonely, tired, fed up, hurt, rejected, or sorry for myself.

Twenty-three years ago I gave up alcohol. Eleven years ago I stopped smoking. In both cases I had to accept it was the first taste of my beloved drug that did the damage. If I resisted the first drink I wouldn't want the next one. If I turned down the first cigarette there wouldn't be a second.

With food it's not so simple because you have to eat. But I do have a few tricks under my belt. Like knowing that processed foods that contain sugars and carbohydrates set me off on a binge.

So for breakfast I have a wheat-free cereal. It tastes like shit but you get used to it. I add soya milk instead of dairy. For lunch, I have rye bread with lettuce, tomato, and cucumber, and a piece of fruit. For dinner I try and have fish and veg and a baked potato and more fruit. At weekends I relax a bit more.

I also swim fifty lengths of my indoor pool and spend five minutes on my Nordic Track. Why am I telling you this?

I weigh 132 pounds and can get into a size 6. Nature would like me to be fifteen pounds heavier. I, on the other hand, dream of being as skinny as the thinnest Spice Girl.

At fifty-seven I can't earn a living on television if I am heavy. Then again, by having a television career I have been able to afford the indoor swimming pool and the Nordic Track.

I can also afford the best restaurants in London and Los Angeles and New York, where I mostly work. But like the pathetic person I am, I mostly watch everyone else enjoying the food while I play with a stupid bit of Dover sole.

I have girlfriends who walk or run three hours a day so they eat what they want. I haven't got time. In any case the exercise I do – less than forty minutes a day – is boring enough.

When I am working full throttle in a television studio some of this regime goes to hell. No, actually it all goes to hell. But the times when I behave myself balance out the times when I don't.

To complete the sad picture I think about my weight constantly. Yes, of course, I am an addictive personality. So how do I cope now I have given up booze, tobacco, and any food remotely tasty? You should see my wardrobe! There is an outfit for every single depressed moment I have ever had.

The author of this book, incidentally, thinks I am wonderful whether I am thin/fat/stylishly dressed or looking like a homeless person. He is brilliant. That's why he is my agent.

David Puttnam

I have watched David progress through life from photographers' agent to film producer to, most recently and happily, a peer of the realm and a great expert on education. He has made a lot of dinner and party rounds in his time, and I still bump into him on the rubber-chicken circuit occasionally. He is as slim now as he was when I first met him in the early 1970s.

David's secret is his wife, Patsy, who has been telling him for years that the appropriate way to eat is "Organic, Vegetarian, Wheatless, Sugarless." The secret of his slim-line figure? A standard diet of:

- grilled tomatoes for breakfast
- smoked salmon for lunch
- pasta with loads of garlic accompanied by a plate of bresaola or prosciutto on the side.

Erica Jong

Erica Jong, friend, client, and famous novelist (*Fear of Flying*), is a kindred spirit. She loves to wine and dine, for preference in far-flung, exotic, and luxurious places. And she needs to watch her weight!

You've inspired me to start my own Obvious Diet. I know that high-protein, low-fat, lots of vegetables but limited fruit works for me so that's what I've embarked on – for the millionth time in my life! Poached eggs and cottage cheese or fruit and cottage cheese for breakfast, fish and salad for lunch, fish and vegetables for dinner, lots of water, lots of Diet Coke and lime, the occasional fresh-fruit sorbet to satisfy my sweet tooth.

My biggest problem is carbohydrate-craving when I'm under stress. Carbs raise the serotonin level in the blood and make me feel less anxious. Also I have no thyroid tissue, as I suffered from Graves' disease – an autoimmune condition in which your own thyroid produces an allergic reaction in the body – when I was nineteen. My thyroid gland was blasted with radiation, so for years I have taken masses of artificial thyroid. This puts me at risk for osteoporosis. As a result, I have to have a diet rich in cottage cheese, broccoli, orange juice, skimmed milk, goat cheese, yogurt, and the like to compensate for calcium loss produced by synthroid and cytomel – the two forms of thyroid I take daily.

I learned much of this stuff from consulting with excellent nutritionists – which I think is a must for any dieter. We all have different bodily needs and not every diet works for every person.

Alcohol plummets the blood sugar level and causes sweet cravings, so I know that alcohol will sabotage my diet. When I want to lose weight, I can't drink even a little.

I have no recipes because it's been my good fortune in life to live with men who are passionate cooks. I make a fabulous vinaigrette dressing, great guacamole, and wonderful omelettes – but these, alas, are not diet dishes. My role in the kitchen is sous chef to some fabulous man – like Ken Burrows, my darling last husband – or Ed Victor, my darling last agent.

Mel Brooks and Anne Bancroft

Mel Brooks and Anne Bancroft are legends individually and as a couple. They both eat healthily and sensibly. You might think that given Mel's origins, he would be wolfing down tons of pastrami sandwiches and pot roast with kasha. Not a bit of it!

We eat very little fat, which cuts out sweets as well because candy and sweets in general are loaded with fats – especially cakes, cookies, and pies.

We try to eat small amounts of animal protein – we are Pritikin-trained. We went there to lower our cholesterol and learned a great deal about health and nutrition. We try to stick to their guidelines – 5 or so helpings of fruits and 5 of vegetables a day – not always easy to do. We try for at least one dark green leafy vegetable among the five. If we have bread with meals, it is always whole grain, either wheat or rye, *never white*. If we have a treat, say a piece of chocolate, it is always dark (less sugar and milk). Our weights are good. We walk for about 40 minutes a day whenever possible – and we keep our upper bodies in good shape by having a terrible fistfight every day (don't take that seriously, please).

Koo Stark

As one of the great beauties of our time, Koo needs to be careful about what she eats, especially since she constantly zooms around the globe attending glamorous events. She is the only one of my friends who has a winter and a summer diet – just like a wardrobe!

Winter Diet (Oh woe is me) Starbucks skinny vanilla latte, Hershey Kisses, old-fashioned porridge oats with maple syrup, lentil soup with carrots, and rhubarb crumble with lashings of custard. Papaya and mango (to remind me that the sun is shining somewhere). Osso buco or champagne risotto with generous shavings of white truffle (yummy). To keep up my spirits, Laurent Perrier rosé champagne when I am on a budget, if no budget, then Cristal. Claret is comforting. Being a visual person, I balance the cold gray winter tones with cheery pink and cream-colored foods.

Summer Diet (Get real, is that me in the mirror? How disgusting!) Time to pin the rules on the fridge door. *Don't* mix protein and carbohydrates; fruit is a separate meal eaten 45 minutes before any other foods. Anything you drink, apart from water, is food.

Don't even mention dairy.

Had to make a mad dash for the kitchen, did a stand-up gorge, head in fridge. How does Nigella Lawson do it? I attacked broccoli and green beans in special sauce (as my daughter calls it) and polished off the whole lot. Summer colors are green to rest the eyes from long hours of unaccustomed sunlight, and red for energy – red cherries, red berries, red apples, and Campari and tonic with a twist of orange for the sunset. Crunchiness and smell are also important. Nothing worse than a flaccid lettuce.

I once did a Cordon Bleu cooking course, right after I got married, in a vain attempt to stay married. I put on 14 pounds, stopped burning the toast, cooked endless dinner parties for eight, and got divorced. I did learn two useful things though: how to cook a delicious roast chicken, and if you want to stay slim, feel well, and have energy, eat anything but *follow the Hay System*. Food combining does work and requires very little self-discipline.

Special Sauce

This can be used for dressing salad or as a marinade.

3 tablespoons olive oil

1 tablespoon tamari or shoyu

juice of half a lime

Combine ingredients.

Idiot's Roast Chicken

1 organic chicken

1 stick butter

handful of fresh tarragon

Preheat the oven to 350°F.

Wash chicken, smear butter lightly around roasting pan, put rest of butter in chicken, squish fresh tarragon to release odor of herb, shove into chicken. Shove into the oven, forget about it for 2$\frac{1}{2}$ hours. Take out and leave to stand with aluminum foil over the top to prevent breast from drying out.

Larry King

Larry's the prime mover of CNN and a man constantly on the move. Like Anne Robinson, his face (and figure) are his fortune, so he is careful about how he eats. Having eaten with him, I would say "very careful." As you will see from his notes ...

1. If it looks like it's wrong to eat from a health stand point, it is!
2. Everything in moderation.
3. Avoid whole milk at all costs.
4. Fruit and vegetables are always right.

Tuna Salad

(Delish, healthy, and filling)
Tuna fish right out of the can, diced,
and mixed with tomatoes, lettuce, and
onions, chopped fine, and dressed
with a light amount of olive oil.

Sir Ranulph Fiennes

As everybody knows, my client Ran Fiennes is one of the fittest men in the world. So, naturally, his diet has evolved to cater to the extraordinary demands he puts on his body. Read his wonderful book *Fit for Life,* in which you will find many excellent diet tips, and then enjoy his reward for good behavior!

Fifth Day Heaven

(A recipe after four days of dieting without slip-ups)

Take one Milky Way bar (not two!) and cut it into slices, as you would a loaf of bread. Stir these in a pan with three cups of semi-skimmed milk over low heat. Add a teaspoon of instant coffee. Stir until it forms a rich sauce. Pour this over the ice cream of your choice. Realize that you cannot repeat this gorgeous experience until you've been good for another four whole days.

Sidney Sheldon

Sidney, one of the world's most famous and popular novelists, has a lifestyle to match. Hence his simple rules to stay slim despite his social obligations ...

1. Do not eat in the kitchen.
2. Smaller portions are preferable – and take a second portion if still hungry.
3. Do not focus on food on occasions that don't warrant it.

As a favorite meal, hamburgers made from minced steak with all the fat trimmed beforehand, with unfancy mustard and ketchup, and thin bread instead of rolls.

There is no greater luxury than freshly squeezed juice.

Do not eat in the kitchen.

Tina Brown

Tina Brown leads a professional and social life as busy and hectic as anyone I know ... myself included! But she always looks trim and immaculate. That is no accident; she works hard at it, and her observations set out below on how she survives American-size portions make fascinating reading.

Living in the U.S., I have found that my downfall is portion size. Little by little I got used to accepting plates laden with three times the amount that's necessary, which is the American way, no matter what you tell the waiter. Combine this with working at a killer pace which leaves no time for menu planning and the stage for disaster is set. I gained ten pounds without even noticing it! My willpower seemed to have collapsed. So I took myself off for a week to the Golden Door Spa in San Diego – where I haven't been since the birth of my first child turned me into a colossus – and they got me back in shape.

The trip to the Door was brilliant, not because I lost more than a few pounds, but because it re-educated me. For over a year I had been doing crash three-day diets and fad diets to get myself into a particular dress on a particular day and then returning to my old bad habits. At the Golden Door I was reminded there is no substitute for the old-fashioned way. Call it the Push Diet. I had to learn all over again to push my plate away. Portion-wise, the easiest thing for me to remember was that the meat or fish on my plate should be NO BIGGER THAN A DECK OF CARDS and the rest of the plate evenly divided between a small serving of vegetables and one of pasta or potatoes.

My mistake had been to try and cut out some foods, like pasta, altogether and then eat too much protein or fruit. Even fruit can be fattening when you eat an apple between every meal and keep snacking on grapes. Now I have trained myself to cut the portion size. In restaurants I ask for a half portion of Dover sole; a half portion of chicken. The notion of being served with too much and leaving half doesn't work for me. Absent-mindedly, I find myself polishing it off and then realize it too late. Instead of snacking on a whole apple I cut an orange into thin slices, as

I have trained myself to cut the portion size. ... After two weeks my stomach had shrunk.

you might slice a lemon for a drink, and take two at a time throughout the day.

After two weeks my stomach had shrunk, and when I forgot to ask for only two scrambled egg whites and – in true American form – I was brought a heaped plate of six scrambled eggs, I found I couldn't eat them and didn't want to – and the pounds have continued to roll off.

Ken Follett

Ken Follett is one of the world's best-selling novelists – and has a lifestyle to match that position. He also sometimes has to play a "Dennis Thatcher" role to his politician wife, Barbara Follett, MP. So there are perils aplenty in terms of eating – or drinking – too much.

Ken Follett's 3-Step Diet

1. Don't eat breakfast.
2. Don't eat lunch.
3. Don't eat dinner.

If you follow this diet you are sure to lose weight!

If hunger overwhelms you between these missed meals, you can:

1. Have a cup of tea.
2. Have a cappuccino.
3. Eat apples.

Some other useful tips:

1. Never eat when you're not hungry, no matter how impolite you feel. (Politicians cannot follow

this advice, they always have to have a second piece of sponge cake.)

2. Never eat anything you don't like, even if it's good for you. This applies especially to vege-tables.

3. Drink plenty of wine. It contains the only truly worthwhile calories.

Finally, a psychological tip:

When you take your clothes off, do you want her to see Falstaff or Brad Pitt?

When you take your clothes off, do you want her to see Falstaff or Brad Pitt?

Art Cooper

Art Cooper has been the very successful editor of *GQ* magazine for 19 years, which any observer of the shark-infested magazine scene will tell you is an eternity. Like anyone else in his position, he has to navigate his way through too many breakfasts, lunches, dinners, and cocktail parties. What follows is a stirring account of how Art finally got religion about his eating habits (and simultaneously sorted out his suit size!).

The Testimonial

It was providential, that day last January when I met Ed Victor for lunch at the Ivy in London. Ed was sleek and bespoke. I was well on my way to Marlon Brandoland. My suit size, once 40, was approaching 50. I had to inhale deeply to fasten my hotel robe or buckle the airplane seatbelt. Ed spoke about his own weight loss and gave me a copy of *The Obvious Diet,* which had just been published in England. I read it and pledged that I, too, would lose 50 pounds in six months. Two months later, I have dropped 30 pounds and four suit sizes. A couple of times I have been mistaken for Sean Connery. Surely one day Ed Victor will be escorted to a comfortable place at God's table.

The Tips

- If an incorrigible maitre d', aware you are dieting, serves you a complimentary Grand Marnier soufflé, it is perfectly acceptable to break all fingers on his serving hand.

- Whenever you are tempted to have that third glass of wine, remember how Orson Welles looked in his later years.

- Before attending cocktail or book parties, I stuff my pockets with slices of radish and cucumber and baby carrots to nibble on instead of those fattening canapés. It is well worth the pressing bills for all those damp suits.

- The two most underrated cocktails in the world are a spicy Virgin Mary and a chilled cranberry juice.

- Bananas are the most satisfying food on earth. I eat one each morning for breakfast and one before attending a dinner party at someone's home.

- Mel Brooks, who offers some tips of his own, is the funniest man I have ever met. We once had a delightful lunch of hot pastrami sandwiches at a Beverly Hills deli. Never, ever eat hot pastrami.

Rose Gray and Ruthie Rogers

Rose and Ruthie are the well-known proprietor-chefs of the world-famous River Cafe in London, and the authors of four groundbreaking (and best-selling) cookbooks. If ever there were two people who could casually put on weight in the course of their jobs, Rose and Ruth are at constant risk, surrounded as they are by the most delicious food they create every day in their kitchen. Yet, as you will see, they both eat carefully and stay slim and trim.

Our whole lives are centered around food – eating and cooking. Our kind of work means that we need plenty of energy to feel fit and keep well. The food we love to eat and cook is seasonal, simple Italian.

We both start the day with an interesting breakfast. Sometimes mangoes or melons and freshly squeezed juices, sometimes a light bruschetta – perhaps with olive oil, fresh tomatoes, or salted anchovies. We both love fresh mint tea or lapsang souchong. During the day we stick to fresh, wild fish, and eat red meat rarely. Every day we eat many delicious seasonal vegetables and salads, using olive oil and fresh lemon juice as a dressing.

We prefer to add red or green chilis and lots of herbs, rather than using sauces.

Our advice is to eat small portions of beautifully prepared and carefully considered food. We don't deny ourselves anything, including desserts – we just eat less of them. Also, we enjoy drinking delicious Italian red wines whenever possible.

Our advice is to eat small portions of beautifully prepared and carefully considered food.

Marie Helvin

What can anyone say about Marie Helvin's heavenly looks? She remains one of London's (and the world's) great beauties, and has been so for many years. She has an ageless beauty, and works hard to keep herself in shape, as you will see from her cunning diet tips.

Tips When Dieting

- Drink lots of pure (not sparkling) water.

- Avoid alcohol. If you must have a drink when dieting, have one glass of white wine with lots of ice.

- Have a plate of steamed vegetables as a main meal each day. Squeeze some lemon juice on them, and add a dash of the best-quality olive oil, plus sea salt and masses of cracked black pepper. I have this dish even when I am not dieting. You can also order it in most good restaurants, even if it is not on the menu – but make sure they do not add butter! Almost all vegetables are delicious raw (everything from artichokes to zucchini – but not eggplant!). If you eat mainly vegetables and fruit on your diet, not only will you lose weight, but it will also help to detox your body.

- Forget about all sauces when you are on a diet. Become accustomed to using fresh lemon or lime juice. I make a delicious diet sauce with natural yogurt (not Greek), fresh lemon juice, and masses of fresh herbs and garlic. I use this on my salad or on fish, or even as a dip for crudités.

- Forget about desserts when you are on a diet. Have fresh fruit instead, and eat the skin as well, if you can. Experiment with textures by freezing peeled fruit and then, before eating, puree into a slush. You can mix the fruit, but do not add sugar or cream. Also, limit your intake of fruit; just because it is healthy does not mean you can eat unlimited amounts of it. During the summer, I freeze lots of different types of fruit to eat as a snack. Sliced pineapple is very good, also extra-large seedless grapes, bananas, etc. (but not citrus!). Either eat straight from the freezer or purée into a slush.

- Invest in a juicer and experiment with fresh vegetables or fruit juices instead of a meal. Use your imagination. Learn to cut, chop, slice, grate, julienne, shred, and purée your veg and fruit. It is quite amazing how the flavors can change, just through the cutting process!

- Invest in an "air-popper" popcorn maker, which uses only hot air, with no oil or butter. Make bowls of popcorn and eat as a snack. Sprinkle lightly with water and then shake some low-sodium vegetable powder on it.

- Go on a fruit fast for one day every once in a while. Eat only one type of fruit (but avoid citrus) all day, including the skin if you can. Eat as much as you like. In the winter, apples or pears are good. In summer, try watermelon or grapes.

- Do not eat when you are depressed. Incorporate some of your diet plan into your everyday life after the dieting is over. It is *not* necessary to eat three meals a day!

Brown Rice

Brown rice is full of B vitamins and fiber. It can be broken down and digested easily and quickly, and its incredible absorption means it will soak up toxins released in your gut. Try a meal of brown rice with steamed broccoli, finely chopped scallions, freshly peeled and finely chopped ginger, and crushed garlic. Toss with the best olive oil and fresh lemon juice.

Japanese Rice

Cook the rice according to package instructions. When done, add soy or tamari sauce to taste. Cover the pot and let the rice absorb this flavor. When the rice is cool put into a plastic container that will hold all ingredients. Add tuna. Add dried seaweed cut with scissors or torn (try the seaweed typically used for sushi – not the type with added sugar). Toss all together. Add a little more soy if necessary. Then add chili flakes, mix well, and keep in the fridge. This is an extremely low-fat Japanese-style dish. I eat it cold with some steamed veg on the side as a main meal.

brown rice

Japanese soy sauce or tamari

can of tuna chunks in water

dried seaweed

chili flakes

Swedish Broth

Bring the water to the boil. Clean but do not peel vegetables, and slice. Add vegetables and parsley to boiling water and season with garlic and herbs. Cook for one hour. Strain and drink the juice as a soup. This broth is high in potassium, which helps to accelerate the elimination of uric acid and other inorganic acids from the body. I use this broth when I am on a non-fast detox.

16 cups water

3 lb potatoes, unpeeled

3 carrots, unpeeled

1 leek with outer leaves

1 onion, unpeeled

1 big bunch parsley

garlic and herbs to taste

Andrew Lloyd Webber

If ever someone could be said to "need no introduction," it is Andrew. Arguably the most popular contemporary composer – the Puccini of our times – he is also a well-known aficionado of good food and good wine, as evidenced by the delightful restaurant column he wrote for the *Telegraph* for some years.

Fabulous Tomato Sauce

This isn't just a fabulous dieter's recipe, it's a fabulous recipe ... period. It can be served with poached scallops or shrimp or any poached non-oily white fish, indeed with any combination of the above. It can also be served hot or cold. The key to this sauce is the quality of the tomatoes therein. The best tomatoes for the dish are the sweet cherry variety, preferably from the southern Mediterranean.

Press through a sieve as many tomatoes as you need for the required quantity of sauce. Keep the watery juices and discard the pulp, skin, and seeds. Clarify the tomato juice by bringing it to a boil and straining it into another pan, repeating this process half a dozen times. You should by

now have a juice of serious intensity and sweetness. If you have been unable to obtain tomatoes
with a really strong flavor, sieve a sun-dried
tomato into the juice before you begin the clarify-
ing process.

You can serve the sauce with the seafood either
hot or cold – you will probably want to stay on your
diet for good! If you want an infallible crowd-
pleaser that also looks sensational, serve the
sauce cold, poured around the white meat of
scallops topped with a small spoonful of caviar.

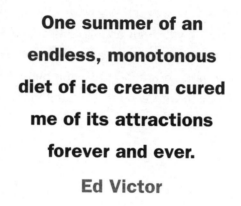

One summer of an endless, monotonous diet of ice cream cured me of its attractions forever and ever.

Ed Victor

CHAPTER NINE

My Obvious Recipes

This chapter is a selection of my own personal Obvious Diet recipes, taken from the cookbooks that have been favorite kitchen-shelf companions over the years. Though they are not necessarily the recipes that first caught my eye when I originally acquired the books, they are the kind of recipes that fit in with my own Obvious Diet. In other words, they provide a kind of safety net of things I know I like, can eat, and still stay trim and healthy. This is an unashamedly biased selection, based on my own tastes alone. One or two of these recipes might not strictly/absolutely/completely adhere to my rules, but they are too delicious to be missed. There are always tactics you can employ to make recipes lighter, such as substituting butter with good olive oil (or leaving it out altogether), or using half the sugar in dessert recipes.

Which reminds me, try as I might, I have very few dessert recipes to offer. As I have mentioned, I'm a sweet-o-phobe – a man who has always asked for his sauce on the side in case the sauce happens to be a nouveau fruit coulis – so I can provide little solace for the inveterate dessert eater.

Incidentally, the last shard of any vestigial sweet tooth I might have possessed disappeared when I was nineteen years old. Until then, the only dessert that remotely interested me was ice cream – perhaps a result of the long, hot summer nights in New York City, where I grew up, punctuated by the ringing of bells on the Good Humor man's truck. At the start of the summer break after my sophomore year at Dartmouth College, I got a job as an ice-cream-truck driver – but I worked for an outfit called Bungalow Bar, the bitter rival of Good Humor. All day long, I cruised the streets in my truck, which had a red shingle roof and white picket fences for doors. I wore a white uniform and had a Sam Browne belt with a change-making machine attached. And I did my best to outwit my opponent, the Good Humor man, by working much, much harder and longer than he did. Thus, obsessed as I was by making money (my first taste of earning a living through commission!), I

Try as I might, I have very few dessert recipes to offer.

never stopped to eat – preferring, instead, to live off the goodies stashed in my truck. One summer of an endless, monotonous diet of ice cream cured me of its attractions forever and ever.

My advice to all you people in thrall to sugar cravings would be that when you feel that sugar need, find and eat some delicious fruit, something that is in season and ripe with sweetness to give you the sugar kick and take you through the danger. Note the in-season part – if you try and wean yourself off sweet treats with tasteless forced fruit that has traveled halfway around the world, your reeducation is going to be harder than Eliza Doolittle's. Now is the moment to go to your local health food store and buy some of the less-than-perfect-looking produce on their shelves. You're looking for taste and sweetness, not perfect external beauty. Stewed fruit makes another excellent and healthy dessert or emergency snack food – my Italian daughter-in-law swears by apples and pears lightly stewed with raisins, with maybe just a drop of Marsala wine as it cooks. Once again, you the dieter have to take responsibility. Do as I have done below. Go to your favorite cookbooks, vegetarian, and alternative cookbooks, and see what you can find in recipes that have no sugar, little sugar, honey instead of sugar ... you already know the obvious ways to achieve what you want to achieve.

A Word about Chicken Soup

Growing up in a Jewish home in Brooklyn, I am of the firm belief that chicken soup is, indeed, a panacea for whatever ails you. There is a story (probably apocryphal, but who cares?) that, many years ago, the Weizmann Institute of Science in Rehovoth, Israel, proved scientifically that chicken soup "cured" colds and flu. Whether or not it actually does, I find it delicious. And, if properly configured, it can be part of The Obvious Diet. For good measure, I've added another two versions of chicken soup, one as made for me by my great friend and exceptional photographer Eve Arnold, the other a tasty version from Nigella Lawson's recent book *Nigella Bites*.

My mother, Lydia, was a great, but by no means sophisticated, cook. So the idea of *al dente* vegetables never reached her. I honor her sensibility in this recipe by not adding the vegetables later or removing them sooner. I just let them cook with the chicken until they are overdone and squishy, and eat them as a side dish with the boiled chicken pieces.

My Mother's Chicken Soup

Put the chicken (plus feet and giblets, if you have them) in a large pot and cover with cold water. Bring to a rolling boil, then skim off froth with a metal spoon.

Add vegetables (quantities are never exact – use your judgment), salt and peppercorns, and a peeled and quartered clove of garlic if you like. Add a good handful of parsley (with the stems left on).

Turn down heat and simmer until the chicken is tender and cooked through (around 2 hours).

Remove the chicken and vegetables. The ideal thing is to let it stand until cool, then skim any fat from the top with a metal spoon. It's even tastier – and more effective? – the next day (and then the day after that), so make large quantities. The boiled chicken makes a delicious main course, but remember to take the skin off!

1 large boiling fowl (regular roasting chickens will NOT do), cut into four pieces – hopefully the butcher can provide you with the feet and the giblets.

carrots

onions

leeks

sea or kosher salt

black peppercorns

garlic (optional)

parsley

Eve Arnold's Special Chicken Soup for Ed

Eve ends her recipe with the words "bon appetit!" and an apology that the recipe has no exact measurements. "Just improvise" is her advice.

One dark, depressing midwinter's day in London, I heard that my friend and agent, Ed Victor, was in bed with a croaking cold. So I decided to take the afternoon off and make him a chicken soup.

It was in the '70s when local merchants were still making deliveries. First I called the poulterer and discussed the chicken with him. He suggested that instead of the classic big fat hen, I use a pullet (a young bird a year old). He said he would cut it into eight pieces and then I was on my own.

Next I called the greengrocer and asked which vegetables they had. They told me and I ordered. What arrived were the following: parsnips, carrots, green and red peppers, celery, sweet potatoes, onions, and a lemon. From here on in I improvised.

I wiped the pullet clean, put it in the pot with the following: 2 peppers cut in

quarters, 2 whole carrots, 1 large onion
(into which I inserted cloves), 1 whole
sweet potato, 1 parsnip, and 4 stalks of
celery.

I covered the whole thing with boiling
water and then simmered the lot until
the pullet was tender – I think it was
¾ of an hour; it could have been longer.

When the bird was tender and the
vegetables almost disintegrated, I
removed the vegetables and discarded
them, then I skinned the chicken,
shredded it into edible bits, and put the
shredded chicken back in the stock.

Next I diced fresh red and green
peppers, carrots, sweet potatoes,
parsnips, and celery. To these I added
some frozen peas, a diced potato, the
juice of ½ a lemon, and salt and pepper
to taste, and added them to the soup.
This I cooked until the vegetables were
al dente.

Ed still remembers this soup twenty-five
years later – as do I that nasty day when
I enjoyed making it.

Nigella Lawson's Chicken Soup

(minus Kneidlach dumplings –
from *Nigella Bites*)

Serves 4 (or 8 Gentiles)
2 small or 1 large boiling chicken
1 unpeeled onion, halved
1 stalk celery
2 carrots, peeled and cut in chunks
a few sprigs of parsley
a few peppercorns
2 bay leaves
1 tablespoon salt

Put all the ingredients in a large stockpot, cover abundantly with water, and bring to the boil. Skim to remove all the gray scum that will float to the surface, then let cook at a simmer for about 3 hours (if you have a boiling chicken; if it's a roaster, it should be half that, though for that real extra flavor take the flesh off the carcass and slip the carcass back in for another good long stint). Just keep tasting. When the broth tastes golden and chickeny, it's ready. Remove the chicken and, if you like, leave the soup to get cold so you can remove any fat that collects on the surface. That way you accrue some schmalz, too.

Reheat the stock, and serve it as a plain soup, or add a few carrot sticks – from about 2 carrots, say – and cook in the soup, adding some torn-up pieces of chicken to warm through at the end. I like to add freshly chopped parsley.

Vegetable Soup with Vermicelli

(from *The Martha Stewart Cookbook*)

In a heavy 5–6 quart casserole, sauté the onions in the oil until soft. Add the garlic, peppers, and carrots. Cook for 5 minutes. Add the potatoes and stock and simmer until potatoes are almost tender.

Add the green beans and zucchini and simmer for 5 minutes. Stir in the vermicelli and continue cooking until the vermicelli is *al dente*. Season with salt and pepper and sprinkle with parsley.

Serve piping hot.

(*Note* I enjoy this without the vermicelli – you could too!)

Serves 10

2 large onions, sliced thin

$1/2$ cup olive oil

2 garlic cloves, crushed

2 large red peppers, cut into 1 x $1^1/4$-in. strips

1 lb carrots, peeled and cut into $1/2$-in. cubes

$1^1/2$ lb potatoes, cut into $1/4$-in. cubes

7 cups chicken stock

2 lb green beans, cut into 1-in. pieces

3 small zucchini, cut lengthwise into 1-in. pieces

$1/2$ lb vermicelli

coarse kosher or sea salt and freshly ground black pepper to taste

heaping $1/4$ cup chopped fresh flat-leaf parsley

Ceviche of Sea Bass

(from *Le Dome at Home*)

Makes a starter for 12

3 lb fresh sea bass
fillets

8 large tomatoes, diced

2 large cucumbers,
diced

6 large red onions, diced

6 heaping tablespoons
chopped cilantro

3 heaping tablespoons
chopped fresh parsley

juice of 6 lemons

salt and pepper to taste

Cut the sea bass into $\frac{1}{2}$-inch-square pieces and place them in a bowl. Mix in all the remaining ingredients (keep a little salt, pepper, and lemon juice aside to adjust the flavor later). Add just enough water to cover everything. Cover and marinate in the refrigerator for at least 3 hours.

Remove the ceviche from the refrigerator just before serving. Adjust the taste by adding additional salt, pepper, and lemon juice. Serve the ceviche in individual bowls.

Oven-Baked Fillet of Sea Bass

(from *Le Dome at Home*)

Preheat the oven to 350°F.

Using some of the olive oil, brush a piece of parchment paper large enough to wrap the fish in. Rub the paper with the garlic clove. Spread the spinach leaves over the paper and place the bass in the center. Sprinkle the fish with salt and pepper.

Arrange the fennel, thyme, bay leaves, oregano, tomatoes, shallots, and lemon slices on top of the fish. Sprinkle with the remaining olive oil and the white wine. Wrap the paper around the bass to prevent the juices and steam from escaping. Place the fish on a baking sheet and put it in the preheated oven. Bake for 25 minutes.

To serve, transfer the wrapped fillet to a serving platter. Cut the paper at the table so your guests can enjoy the escaping aromas.

Serves 6

$1/2$ **cup extra virgin olive oil**

1 clove garlic, cut in half

18 whole spinach leaves, cleaned

1 whole sea bass, approximately 3 lb, filleted

salt and pepper to taste

6 sprigs fennel

6 sprigs fresh thyme

3 bay leaves

1 teaspoon chopped fresh oregano

6 tomato slices

2 shallots, chopped

lemon slices

3 tablespoons dry white wine

Grilled Marinated Filet Mignon of Tuna

(from *The Union Square Café Cookbook*)

Serves 4

Marinade

2 cups teriyaki sauce

1/2 cup dry sherry

1/4 cup finely chopped fresh ginger

1/2 bunch scallions, chopped

2 garlic cloves, thinly sliced

1/2 teaspoon cayenne

2 teaspoons freshly ground black pepper

juice of 2 lemons

Tuna

4 tuna steaks, 8 to 10 ounces each, cut into 3-inch cubes

2 tablespoons olive oil

1/4 cup Japanese pickled ginger

The biggest trick to make this taste like the dish in our restaurant is to convince your fishmonger to cut the tuna steaks into 3-inch cubes, 8 to 10 ounces each, from the reddest possible tuna, so they look just like filet mignon steaks.

Combine all the marinade ingredients in a bowl large enough to hold the tuna. Place the tuna steaks in the marinade and refrigerate for 3 hours, turning every hour.

Thirty minutes before cooking, drain the tuna and bring to room temperature. Preheat a grill, grill pan, or outdoor barbecue to very hot.

Brush the tuna with the olive oil. Grill the steaks for 1 to 2 minutes on each of their six sides. The outside of the tuna should be nicely charred and the center should be barely warm and quite rare. Cooked this way, the tuna will remain moist and flavorful.

Top each steak with pickled ginger and serve.

Rombo con Rosmarino al Sale

Whole Turbot with Rosemary Baked in
Sea Salt

(from *The Cafe Cookbook*)

*Buy a fresh turbot that is not thick
with roe and still has sea slime on its
skin. Have the fishmonger remove only
the gut.*

Preheat the oven to 425°F.

Use a large baking sheet that will snugly
hold the turbot. Cover the bottom with a
layer of salt and place the turbot on the
salt. Push the rosemary into the cavity
and completely cover the fish with the
remainder of the salt, about ¾ inch
thick. Do not worry if the head and tail
protrude. Sprinkle the surface of the
salt with a little water – use a few tablespoons.

Place in the preheated oven and bake
for 25 to 35 minutes. After 20 minutes,
test by inserting a skewer into the
center of the fish. If the skewer is warm,
the turbot is cooked.

Allow to cool for 5 minutes, then crack
open the salt crust. Carefully remove as

Serves 6

**1 turbot with head and
tail intact, about 6 to 7
lb**

**7 to 8 lb natural coarse
sea salt**

1 bunch fresh rosemary

**freshly ground black
pepper**

**balsamic vinegar (aged
and thick)**

extra virgin olive oil

3 lemons

much of the salt as possible. You will find the thick skin of the turbot will stick to the salt.

Serve at room temperature, with coarsely ground black pepper, a few dribbles of balsamic vinegar, extra virgin olive oil, and a half lemon.

Branzino Ripieno d'Erbe

Sea Bass Slashed and Stuffed with Herbs

(from *The Cafe Cookbook*)

Preheat the grill or griddle. It must be very hot and clean.

Make ½-inch-deep slashes across the width of the whole sea bass at 2½-inch intervals. Slash the skin side of the fillets in the same way. Season the fish with salt and pepper. Mix the herbs together and then push as much of this mixture into the slashes as you can.

Place the whole fish on the grill and do not turn over until it is completely seared. Turn over when the fish comes away easily. When seared on both sides, reduce the heat and continue grilling until the fish is cooked. Alternatively, grill the fillets, skin side down first, on the grill.

Mix the juice of 1 of the lemons with the olive oil, and pour over the grilled fish, then scatter any remaining herbs over. Serve with lemon wedges.

Serves 6

1 sea bass, about 7 to 8 lb in weight, scaled and cleaned, or

6 to 7 oz individual sea bass fillets

sea salt and freshly ground black pepper

2 tablespoons each of fresh marjoram, fresh basil or mint, and fresh green fennel or dill, roughly chopped

3 lemons

3½ oz extra virgin olive oil

Sogliola al Forno con Origano e Alloro

Roasted Dover Sole with Oregano and Bay

(from *The Cafe Cookbook*)

Serves 6

extra virgin olive oil

6 lemons

24 dried bay leaves

1/4 cup dried wild oregano

6 whole Dover sole, weighing about 12 to 14 oz each, scaled and cleaned

sea salt and coarsely ground black pepper

Preheat the oven to 450°F. Brush 2 large baking sheets with olive oil. Slice 2 of the lemons into fine discs 1/16 inch thick. Scatter half the bay leaves, a few of the lemon slices, and some oregano on the bottom of the pans. Place the soles on top, season generously, then scatter the remaining oregano, bay leaves, and lemon slices on top of the fish to cover them. Drizzle generously with olive oil and bake in the preheated oven for 15 to 20 minutes. Test, using the point of a sharp knife down the center of the thickest part of the sole. If cooked, the flesh should just be coming away from the bone.

Remove the sole from the pans. Place the pans with the herbs and fish juices over a medium heat and deglaze with the juice from 3 of the remaining lemons. Serve each sole with some of this sauce, the herb leaves, and lemon wedges cut from the remaining lemon.

Sea Bass Baked with Mussels and Shrimp

(from *The East Hampton Cookbook*)

Preheat the oven to 375°F.

Line a grill pan (or baking dish large enough to hold the fish) with heavy-duty aluminum foil. Set aside.

Wash and dry the fish, then season with salt and pepper. Stuff with tarragon and parsley and set aside.

Melt the butter (or put the olive oil) in the grill pan; add chopped onions, stir to coat them, and bake about 10 minutes, or until soft. Add sliced mushrooms and wine, stir, and lay fish on top. Bake 25 minutes.

Put mussels around fish, baste both, and bake 10 minutes longer. Add shrimp, baste everything again, and bake another 10 minutes. At the end of the 45 minutes cooking time the mussels will be open, the shrimp pink, and the fish baked through. (If using a larger fish, increase the initial baking time accordingly.)

Serves 6

1 sea bass, 5 lb whole, cleaned and gutted, head and tail left on

salt and fresh pepper

2 to 3 sprigs fresh tarragon or $^1/_2$ teaspoon dried

several parsley sprigs

6 tablespoons butter (as always, good olive oil can be substituted)

2 medium onions, chopped

4 oz mushrooms, sliced

$^3/_4$ to 1 cup white wine

8 oz mussels, debearded and scrubbed

8 oz raw shrimp, shelled and deveined

1 heaping tablespoon fresh chopped parsley

3 lemons, cut in half

Cover the body of the fish with chopped parsley and serve right in the grill pan, garnished with lemon halves.

(*Note* Any firm-fleshed whole white fish can be substituted with equally good results.)

Calamari ai Ferri con Peperoncini

Grilled Squid with Chilis

(from *The Rogers Gray Italian Country Cookbook*)

Clean the squid by cutting the body open to make a flat piece. Scrape out the guts, keeping the tentacles in their bunches but removing the eyes and mouth.

Using a serrated knife, score the inner side of the flattened squid body with parallel lines $1/2$ inch apart, and then equally apart the other way to make cross-hatching.

To make the sauce, put the chopped chilis in a bowl and cover with about 1 inch of the oil. Season with salt and pepper.

Place the squid (including the tentacles) scored side down on a very hot grill, season with salt and pepper, and grill for 1 to 2 minutes. Turn the squid pieces over; they will immediately curl up, by which time they will be cooked.

Toss the arugula in the Oil and Lemon Dressing. Arrange a squid body and tentacles on each plate with some of the arugula. Place a little of the chili sauce on the squid and serve with lemon quarters.

Serves 6

6 medium squid, no bigger than your hand

Sauce

12 large fresh red chilis, seeded and very finely chopped

extra virgin olive oil

sea salt and freshly ground black pepper

To serve

$1/2$ cup Oil and Lemon Dressing (see page 235)

8 oz arugula leaves

3 lemons

Grilled Leg of Lamb

(from James Beard's *American Cookery*)

1 leg of lamb, boned and split

olive oil for grilling

salt and pepper to taste

Marinade

1 bottle red wine

1 tablespoon salt

1 tablespoon crushed peppercorns

1 celery stalk, cut in julienne strips

1 teaspoon thyme

1 onion stuck with two cloves

1 bay leaf, crushed

The leg of lamb should be boned (leaving the shank bone) and split so that it is open and flat, although some spots will be thicker than others. The skin should be removed.

Combine the marinade ingredients. Place the lamb in a very large baking dish or nonreactive pan and coat with the marinade.

Marinate for however long you like, from 3 to 4 hours up to 6 days! Turn the leg each day. The longer you leave it, the gamier the flavor will be.

Remove from the marinade and dry thoroughly. Rub well with oil. Grill cut side down, at least 5 or 6 inches from the source of heat, about 15 minutes. Do not allow it to char. Turn it and grill another 10 to 15 minutes, depending on the thickness of the meat. Gauge it almost as you would a thick steak. Salt and pepper well, using freshly ground pepper. Allow to stand 5 minutes. Carve in diagonal slices across the leg.

(*Note* Although I hate to argue with the late, great Mr. Beard, I have cut his timings, because experience has shown them to be too long, and the meat is overcooked. Also, this recipe is absolutely great on the barbecue and makes a wonderful summer supper served with a simple salad or vegetable dish.)

Grilled Butterflied Leg of Lamb

(from *Fannie Farmer Cookbook*)

A tender lamb steak that may be cooked over coals or under the broiler, offering both a crisp well-done exterior and succulent rare insides. Start to marinate in the afternoon.

Serves 6

1/4 cup olive oil

2 cloves garlic, finely diced

1 teaspoon rosemary, crumbled

1 teaspoon salt

1 teaspoon freshly ground pepper

5-lb leg of lamb, split open and bone removed

Preheat the broiler.

Put the olive oil in a small bowl and add the garlic, rosemary, salt, and pepper. Mix well, and rub mixture all over the lamb. Put the meat on a trivet and cover it lightly with parchment paper. Let stand for 2 to 3 hours before broiling.

Remove the paper and place the lamb on the rack 4 inches below the broiler element. Cook 15 minutes on each side. Test by cutting a small slit in the thickest part – it should be slightly pink inside and nicely browned on top. Slice across the grain on the diagonal, and serve with natural juices.

Hashed Brussels Sprouts with Poppy Seeds and Lemon

(from *The Union Square Café Cookbook*)

This simple recipe has converted lots of sworn brussels sprouts haters into devoted connoisseurs.

Cut the stems from the brussels sprouts and halve each one lengthwise. Slice each half into thin slices, 1/8 inch thick, and toss with the lemon juice in a large bowl.

Heat the olive oil in a frying pan over a high heat almost to the smoking point. Stir in the hashed sprouts with the garlic and poppy seeds. Add the white wine and continue stirring for about 3 minutes, until the sprouts are bright green and barely crunchy. Reduce the heat to low, season with salt and pepper, and cook for 1 additional minute. Transfer to a warm bowl and serve.

Serves 4 to 6 as an accompaniment to a main dish

1 lb large brussels sprouts

juice of 1/2 lemon

2 tablespoons olive oil

2 garlic cloves, peeled and crushed

1 tablespoon poppy seeds

1/4 cup white wine

1/4 teaspoon kosher salt/sea salt

1/8 teaspoon freshly ground black pepper

Sautéed Broccoli di Rape

(from *The Union Square Café Cookbook*)

The natural bitterness of this nutritious green tames as you cook it. Be sure to choose young broccoli rabe that has a vibrant green color, no yellowing in the florets, and tender, not woody stalks.

Serves 4

2 lb broccoli rabe, washed, largest stems discarded

¹/₄ cup extra virgin olive oil, plus more for drizzling

2 teaspoons finely crushed garlic

¹/₃ teaspoon dried red pepper flakes

¹/₂ teaspoon kosher salt/sea salt

¹/₈ teaspoon freshly ground black pepper

³/₄ cup water

4 lemon wedges

Separate the leaves from the florets of the broccoli rabe. Chop the leaves and stems into 3-inch pieces.

In a reasonably large saucepan or frying pan large enough to hold all the greens, combine the olive oil, garlic, and red pepper flakes. Cook over moderately high heat for about 45 seconds to flavor the oil, but do not allow the garlic to brown. Add the broccoli rabe. The pan will be overflowing, but the greens will lose considerable volume during cooking. Continuously toss with tongs to avoid any browning of the greens. It will take 1 to 2 minutes to wilt them.

Add the salt and pepper, toss, and cook for approximately 1 minute longer. Add the water and cook until the greens are tender, 3 to 5 minutes. Garnish with the lemon wedges and a light drizzle of olive oil.

Fava Beans Braised in Milk

(from *River Cafe Cookbook Green*)

Gently heat the olive oil in a medium, thick-bottomed saucepan with a lid. Add the beans and garlic (apart from 1 clove for the bruschetta), and slowly cook together for 10 to 15 minutes or until they become soft. Add the sage, salt, and pepper, and carry on cooking just to allow the sage flavor to penetrate the beans. Pour in the milk, cover the pan, and simmer very gently for 20 minutes, or until the beans have absorbed most of the milk. Taste for seasoning.

Preheat the broiler. Toast the bread on both sides, then rub lightly on one side only with the reserved garlic clove. Spoon the beans and some of their juices over each bruschetta. Scatter over the lemon zest, and drizzle over each a generous amount of extra virgin olive oil.

(Obviously, I omit the bruschetta from this recipe; you don't have to!)

Serves 6

¼ cup olive oil

6 lb fava beans, shelled

1 whole head garlic, divided into cloves, peeled

10 fresh sage leaves, finely minced

sea salt and freshly ground black pepper

5 oz milk

6 slices of sourdough bread

finely grated zest of 1 lemon

extra virgin olive oil

Peas Braised with Scallions

(from *River Cafe Cookbook Green*)

Serves 6
1 lb scallions
6 lb fresh peas
1¹⁄₃ cup chicken stock
¹⁄₄ cup olive oil
sea salt and freshly ground pepper
1 head curly endive
extra virgin olive oil

Trim the scallions, removing the green leafy stalks and the roots. Shell the peas. In a small saucepan, bring the chicken stock to the boil.

In a large, thick-bottomed saucepan, heat the olive oil and gently cook the scallions until they become translucent but not brown. Add the peas, season with salt and pepper, and stir to coat all the peas with the olive oil. Add enough stock to cover the peas generously and cover the mixture with a piece of parchment paper. Reduce the heat as low as possible and cook for 15 minutes or until the scallions are completely tender.

Remove all the outer leaves of the curly endive and discard. Tear the small white leaves into shreds and stir into the peas. Cook for a further few minutes until the endive is wilted. Drizzle with extra virgin olive oil to finish. Serve at room temperature.

Plain Boiled Asparagus

(from *The Way to Cook*, Julia Child)

Once peeled, asparagus is easy to cook. None of that old-fashioned steaming the tips and boiling the butts business because the stalks are tender from end to end.

Lay the asparagus in the boiling salted water, cover the casserole or pan, and watch carefully until water comes back to the boil; immediately uncover it. Boil slowly for 4 to 5 minutes, just until asparagus spears start to bend a little when lifted. Test by eating the butt end of a spear. Asparagus should be just cooked through with a slight crunch. Immediately remove the asparagus from the water.

For 6 servings, 6 to 8 fat spears per person

36 to 48 fine fresh asparagus spears, all the same diameter, and all peeled

2 quarts rapidly boiling water in an oval casserole or large frying pan

1 1/2 teaspoons salt per quart of water

To serve hot: Arrange on a napkin-lined platter to catch moisture; or drain briefly on a clean towel, then arrange on a hot platter or on hot plates.

To serve cold: Drain in one layer on a baking sheet lined with a clean towel and rapidly cool, near an open window if possible. Arrange on a platter or plates.

Suggested accompaniments if serving hot:

Melted butter, hollandaise sauce, lemon-butter sauce, and/or lemon wedges.

(*Note* Dietetic alternatives for serving hot include drizzling with olive oil, lightly seasoning with salt and pepper, sprinkling over a few drops of balsamic vinegar, and then, if you must, dusting with Parmesan shavings.)

Suggested accompaniments if serving cold:

Vinaigrette dressing and its variations, mayonnaise, and/or lemon wedges.

(*Note* If you are seasoning the asparagus with vinaigrette dressing, which should be added at the last minute to preserve the green asparagus color, you may then wish to decorate with strips of red pepper, or spoon over the upper third a mixture of chopped hard-boiled eggs and parsley tossed with a sprinkle of salt.)

Peperoni al Forno con Pomodoro e Acciughe

Baked Peppers with Tomatoes and Anchovies

(from *The Cafe Cookbook*)

Preheat the oven to 350°F.

Halve each pepper lengthwise and remove the core and seeds. Place the peppers in a lightly oiled baking dish, cut side up. Into each half pepper put 3 tomatoes, 2 slivers of garlic, 2 anchovy fillets, a few basil or marjoram leaves, and 3–4 capers. Lightly drizzle the peppers with the remaining olive oil and season with salt and pepper.

Pour about 1¼ cups water into the bottom of the baking dish to prevent the peppers from sticking. Cover the dish tightly with foil. Bake in the preheated oven for 20 minutes, then remove from the oven. Remove the foil, reduce the oven temperature to 250–300°F, and bake for an additional 40 minutes or until the peppers are soft.

Serves 6

3 red and 3 yellow peppers

5 tablespoons olive oil

36 cherry tomatoes

3 garlic cloves, peeled and cut into slivers

24 salted anchovy fillets, rinsed

1 bunch fresh basil or marjoram

4 oz salted capers, rinsed

sea salt and freshly ground pepper

Zucchini Carpaccio

(from *The Cafe Cookbook*)

Use only small young zucchini for this salad.

Serves 6

2 ¼ lb young yellow and green zucchini

8 oz arugula

3 tablespoons extra virgin olive oil

juice of 1 lemon

sea salt and freshly ground black pepper

4 to 6 oz slivers of Parmesan sliced from a single piece

Trim the ends off the zucchini and slice at an angle into thin rounds. Place in a bowl.

Pick through the arugula, discarding any yellow leaves. Snap off the stalks, then wash and dry the leaves thoroughly.

Mix together the olive oil, lemon juice, and salt and pepper, and pour over the zucchini. Mix, then leave to marinate for 5 minutes. Season with salt and pepper.

Divide the arugula leaves among the serving plates. Put the zucchini on top, and then the Parmesan slivers. Add a small amount of freshly ground black pepper, and serve.

Frittata di Zucchini

(from *The Cafe Cookbook*)

Preheat the oven to 400°F.

Trim the zucchini, then cut thinly at an angle. Heat 2 tablespoons of the oil in an ovenproof frying pan. Add the garlic followed by the zucchini slices. When the zucchini are brown on all sides, add most of the basil and salt and pepper to taste. The zucchini should be quite dry; If there is any oil remaining, drain through a sieve and reserve.

Break the eggs into a bowl and beat lightly. Add the zucchini and garlic, reserving 1 tablespoon for the end. Season with salt and pepper.

Cook the frittata in an ovenproof frying pan on a low heat until the egg is almost set, using the reserved oil as well as the further tablespoon if necessary. Just before placing it into the hot oven, spread the rest of the zucchini on top. Remove from the oven and sprinkle with the Parmesan and the remaining basil. Serve.

Serves 6

4 small or 3 medium zucchini

3 tablespoons olive oil

2 garlic cloves, peeled and chopped

1 small bunch fresh basil, leaves picked from the stems and shredded by hand

sea salt and freshly ground black pepper

8 organic eggs

2 oz Parmesan, grated

Cipolle Rosse Ripiene di Timo

Baked Red Onions and Thyme

(from *The Cafe Cookbook*)

Serves 6

12 small red onions, skins left on

4 garlic cloves, peeled and thinly sliced

1 bunch fresh thyme, leaves of 2 sprigs picked from the stems

1½ sticks unsalted butter, softened

sea salt and freshly ground black pepper

5 to 6 oz balsamic vinegar

5 oz red wine

Preheat the oven to 350°F.

Trim the base of each onion. Cut in a deep cross from the top, to about halfway down the onion. Stand the onions in a baking dish and place a couple of slivers of garlic and a small sprig of the thyme in the incisions. Mix the butter with the remaining thyme leaves, salt, and pepper, and put a teaspoonful on top of each onion. Drizzle the balsamic vinegar and red wine over the onions and season again. Cover with aluminum foil and bake in the preheated oven for about 40 minutes or until the onions have softened.

Remove the foil and reduce the oven temperature to 300°F, and continue to cook for another hour, basting frequently. To prevent the balsamic juices from drying up and burning, add 1¼ cups or so of water, or more red wine. Reduce temperature to 250°F and the onions can be roasted for longer. The onions are ready when they are soft and caramelized.

Carciofi in Padella

Artichokes Braised with White Wine

(from *The Rogers Gray Italian Country Cookbook*)

Prepare the artichokes, then rub with a lemon half to prevent discoloring.

In a large heavy saucepan heat 2 tablespoons of the olive oil over a medium heat. Fry the artichokes until they begin to color, then add the thyme and garlic. Season generously with salt and pepper. Stir occasionally.

When the garlic begins to color, add the white wine, the juice from the remaining lemon half, and enough olive oil, about 5 ounces, to cover. Put the lid on, and simmer gently for about 30 minutes, or until the artichokes are tender.

Serves 6

12 small globe artichokes, with stalks, prepared

1 lemon, halved

olive oil

1 bunch fresh thyme, leaves picked from the stems

4 garlic cloves, peeled and thinly sliced

sea salt and freshly ground black pepper

5 oz dry white wine

Peperoni in Padella

Peppers in Olive Oil

(from *The Cafe Cookbook*)

Serves 6

8 large ripe dark red peppers

¼ cup olive oil

sea salt and freshly ground black pepper

3 tablespoons herb wine vinegar

Wash and dry the peppers, then cut in half lengthwise and then in half again and again. Using a small paring knife, remove any white membrane on the inside of the peppers, plus the seeds.

Use a large frying pan or low-sided large saucepan with a lid. Heat half the olive oil and place some of the pepper pieces in one layer. Fry over a medium to high heat with the lid on, turning the pieces over as they begin to color and become soft. Remove with a slotted spoon and keep warm. Repeat with a second layer of peppers, and continue until you have cooked them all. You may have to use extra oil if you fry in more than two batches. Drain off excess oil.

Return all the peppers to the pan, reheat together, and season with salt, pepper, and vinegar.

Carciofi alla Giudea

Deep-Fried Whole Artichokes

(from *The Rogers Gray Italian Country Cookbook*)

This traditional Jewish dish from Rome is stunning in its simplicity and boldness.

Using a small, sharp knife, remove the tougher outer leaves of the artichokes and, if necessary, trim the spikes from the top. Cut the stalks, leaving about 2 inches, and peel.

Using your fingers, gently pry open each artichoke, turn it upside down and, while pressing down with one hand, pull out the leaves with the other. The aim is to open up and flatten the artichoke. Season the opened surface with salt and pepper.

Heat the oil to 350°F in a deep fryer or large, deep saucepan. Plunge two or three artichokes into the hot oil at a time, and fry just until the leaves curl up and become crisp, about 3 to 4 minutes. Drain well on paper towels.

Serve with lemon halves.

Serves 6

12 small globe artichokes with their stalks

sea salt and freshly ground black pepper

sunflower oil for deep frying

3 lemons, halved

Radicchio alla Griglia

Grilled Radicchio

(from *The Rogers Gray Italian Country Cookbook*)

Serves 6

3 medium heads of radicchio

sea salt and freshly ground black pepper

Olive Oil and Vinegar Dressing (see page 236)

1 small bunch fresh marjoram, parsley, or basil

Preheat the grill.

Carefully peel open and separate the whole leaves of radicchio. Place the leaves in a single layer on the grill. Season and turn over immediately just to wilt, not to blacken. Place in an ovenproof dish and pour over the dressing. Turn to coat the leaves, add the herbs, and bake in an oven heated to 350°F for 15 minutes.

Zucchini and Tomatoes

(from *The East Hampton Cookbook*)

Wash the zucchini and cut into 1-inch slices. Sauté onion in olive oil in a frying pan until slightly brown. Stir in garlic and tomatoes and cook 5 minutes longer over medium heat. Add zucchini, salt and pepper to taste, bay leaf, and oregano, and cover and cook gently for 20 to 25 minutes or until tender.

If, after 15 minutes there appears to be a great deal of liquid in the pan, remove cover for the last 5 to 10 minutes of cooking. Taste for seasoning, remove bay leaf, and serve immediately.

Serves 4

4 to 5 medium zucchini

1 small onion, sliced

2 tablespoons olive oil

1 clove garlic, crushed

2 fresh tomatoes, peeled and chopped

1 teaspoon salt

freshly ground pepper

$1/2$ bay leaf

1 teaspoon chopped fresh oregano

Sautéed Zucchini with Herbs and Garlic

(from James Beard's *American Cookery*)

Serves 4

6 to 8 small zucchini, cut in quarters lengthwise

2 to 4 tablespoons olive oil

2 finely chopped garlic cloves

1 teaspoon salt

1 tablespoon, or to taste, chopped fresh basil (or another herb)

¹/₂ teaspoon freshly ground pepper

2 tablespoons chopped flat-leaf parsley

Cut the zucchini in thin strips. Heat the olive oil in a heavy frying pan and add the zucchini strips. Sauté lightly, turning them once or twice, for 5 minutes. Add the garlic, salt, and basil. Cover the pan and simmer about 10 minutes, till the zucchini are just tender to the bite. Add the pepper. Serve in a heated dish with chopped parsley for a garnish.

(*Note* Once again, I have the temerity to recommend an adjustment to Mr. Beard's cooking time. I find that, if you simply turn off the heat after the first 5 minutes and leave the zucchini to sit in the covered pan for about another five minutes, the results are absolutely delicious.)

Salade Niçoise

(from *The Way to Cook*, Julia Child)

Shortly before serving, line a handsome, large, and wide salad bowl or a roomy platter with lettuce leaves, drizzle a little olive oil on them, and dust with a sprinkling of salt. Toss the beans in a mixing bowl with a little of the dressing, and correct seasoning. Drizzle a spoonful or two of the dressing over the tomatoes. Season the tuna lightly with a spoonful or two of dressing. Place the potatoes in the center of the bowl or platter; mound beans at strategic intervals, interspersing them with tomatoes and mounds of tuna. Ring the salad with the eggs, and curl an anchovy on top of each. Spoon a little more vinaigrette over all; scatter on olives, capers, and parsley. Serve as soon as possible.

(*Note* I would personally eliminate the potato salad from this recipe.)

Serves 6 to 8

1 large head of butter lettuce, washed and dried

2 to 3 tablespoons virgin olive oil

salt and ground pepper

1 ½ lb fresh green beans, trimmed, blanched, refreshed in cold water, and dried

²/₃ to 1 cup salad dressing, such as Oil and Lemon Dressing (see page 235)

3 or 4 fine ripe red tomatoes, peeled if you wish, and cored, quartered, and seasoned

8 oz oil-packed tuna, drained and flaked

1 quart French potato salad

8 hard-boiled eggs, halved lengthwise

1 can flat anchovy fillets packed in oil, opened and drained

½ cup black Niçoise-type olives

3 tablespoons capers

¼ cup chopped fresh parsley

Coleslaw

(from *The Way to Cook*, Julia Child)

It is hard to say whether potato salad or coleslaw is America's favorite. Coleslaw goes so well with hamburger, with boiled lobster, with grilled fish, on a picnic – it is certainly one of the great inventions. This is my favorite formula because if there are dieters at the table (including me!) the salad is delicious just with its preliminary flavorings, and you can pass the dressings on the side.

Serves 6 to 8

1 fine fresh hard-headed cabbage weighing about 1 ¹/₂ lb

2 celery stalks, diced

2 carrots, grated

¹/₄ cup diced scallions or mild yellow onion

1 finely diced large green pepper

1 small apple, peeled, cored, and finely diced

1 medium cucumber, peeled, halved lengthwise, seeded, and diced

Remove any wilted outside leaves, wash the cabbage, and shred it. Toss the cabbage in a large mixing bowl with the celery, carrots, scallions, green pepper, apple, cucumber, and parsley. Mix together the mustard, vinegar, salt, and sugar. Toss vegetables with the mustard mixture, caraway or cumin, and seasonings. Toss several times, tasting and adding a little more salt or vinegar if you think it needed. Let stand 20 to 30 minutes to let liquids exude. Toss again and drain.

Before serving, drain again, and correct seasoning. Either toss with the mayonnaise and sour cream mixture or serve as is and pass the sauce separately.

(*Note* This is if you're going for a Treat Meal – it tastes just great without the mayonnaise and sour cream mixture too.)

3 to 4 tablespoons chopped fresh parsley

Preliminary Flavoring

$1/2$ tablespoon Dijon-type prepared mustard

2 tablespoons wine (or cider) vinegar

1 teaspoon salt

1 teaspoon sugar

$1/4$ teaspoon caraway or cumin seeds

$1/4$ teaspoon ground bay leaf (if available)

$1/4$ teaspoon celery seeds

several grinds of fresh pepper

Optional Sauce

$1/3$ cup sour cream mixed with $1/2$ cup mayonnaise, plus more if needed

Insalata Invernale

Winter Salad

(from *The Rogers Gray Italian Country Cookbook*)

Before the flowers form on the dandelion, pick the small center leaves from wild plants.

Serves 6

a handful each of arugula, dandelion, trevise or radicchio, red or white chicory or young spinach, lamb's lettuce

Oil and Lemon Dressing (see opposite)

Wash and pick over the arugula and dandelion leaves. Separate the trevise or radicchio and chicory leaves from their stalks and check for dirt. Mix all the leaves together in a bowl and toss with dressing.

Dressings

(from *The Rogers Gray Italian Country Cookbook*)

These quantities are just a guide. If the oil is very young or the lemon juice mild, you will have to adjust by tasting.

Oil and Lemon Dressing

Combine ingredients; whisk until smooth.

6 tablespoons extra virgin olive oil

2 tablespoons lemon juice

sea salt and freshly ground black pepper

Oil, Lemon, Vinegar, and Garlic Dressing

Combine ingredients; whisk until smooth.

6 tablespoons extra virgin olive oil

1 tablespoon lemon juice

1 tablespoon white/red wine vinegar

1 garlic clove, peeled and crushed with a little sea salt

freshly ground black pepper

Olive Oil and Vinegar Dressing

6 tablespoons extra virgin olive oil

2 to 3 tablespoons red wine or balsamic vinegar

freshly ground black pepper

Combine ingredients; whisk until smooth.

Salsa Verde

(from *The Rogers Gray Italian Country Cookbook*)

1 large bunch flat-leaf parsley

1 bunch fresh basil

handful of fresh mint leaves

3 garlic cloves, peeled

4 oz salted capers, rinsed

4 oz salted anchovies, rinsed

2 tablespoons red wine vinegar

5 tablespoons extra virgin olive oil

1 tablespoon Dijon mustard

sea salt

freshly ground black pepper

If using a food processor, pulse-chop the parsley, basil, mint, garlic, capers, and anchovies until roughly blended. Transfer to a large bowl and add the vinegar. Slowly pour in the olive oil, stirring constantly, and finally add the mustard. Check for seasoning.

This sauce may also be prepared by hand, on a board, preferably using a mezzaluna.

Sauce Vinaigrette

French Dressing

(from *Mastering the Art of French Cooking*)

The basic French dressing of France is a mixture of good wine vinegar, good oil, salt, pepper, fresh green herbs in season, and mustard if you like it. Garlic is employed usually only in southern France. Worcestershire sauce, curry, cheese, and tomato flavorings are not French additions, and sugar is heresy.

The usual proportion of vinegar to oil is one to three, but you should establish your own relationship. Lemon juice or a mixture of lemon and vinegar may be used, and the oil may be a tasteless salad oil, or olive oil. For salads, make the dressing in the empty bowl or a jar, so that all ingredients are well blended and flavored before the salad is mixed with the dressing. And be sure the salad greens are perfectly dry so the dressing will adhere to the leaves. Salad dressings are always best when freshly made. If they stand around for several days they tend to acquire a rancid taste.

For about ¹/₂ cup

¹/₂ to 2 tablespoons good wine vinegar or a mixture of vinegar and lemon juice

¹/₈ teaspoon salt

¹/₄ teaspoon dry mustard (optional)

6 tablespoons salad oil or olive oil

big pinch of pepper

1 to 2 tablespoons green herbs, such as parsley, chives, tarragon, basil; or a pinch of dried herbs (optional)

Beat either the vinegar or lemon juice mixture in a bowl with the salt and optional mustard until the salt is dissolved, then beat in the oil by droplets, and season with pepper, or place all the ingredients in a screw-top jar and shake vigorously to blend thoroughly.

Stir in the optional herbs and correct seasoning just before dressing the salad.

Sauce Ravigote

Vinaigrette with Herbs, Capers, and Onions

(from *Mastering the Art of French Cooking*)

To serve with cold or hot boiled meats

Stir all the ingredients into the
vinaigrette and taste for seasoning.

**1 cup Sauce Vinaigrette
(see page 237)**

**1 teaspoon chopped
capers**

**1 teaspoon very finely
minced shallot or
scallions**

**2 tablespoons minced
fresh green herbs,
parsley, chives, tarragon,
chervil, or parsley only**

Sauce Moutarde

Cold Mustard Sauce with Herbs

(from *Mastering the Art of French Cooking*)

To serve with cold meats and vegetables

2 tablespoons prepared mustard, preferably the strong Dijon type

¹/₃ to ¹/₂ cup olive oil or salad oil

salt and pepper

lemon juice

1 to 2 tablespoons parsley or minced fresh green herbs

Rinse a small mixing bowl in hot water. Add the mustard and beat with a wire whip, adding 3 tablespoons boiling water by droplets.

Again, by droplets, beat in the olive oil to make a thick, creamy sauce.

Beat in salt, pepper, and lemon juice to taste. Then beat in the herbs.

And I'm afraid just a single tasty dessert I'm sometimes tempted to eat ...

Pesche Gratinate con Amaretto

Grilled Peaches with Amaretto

(from *The Rogers Gray Italian Country Cookbook*)

Preheat the oven to 375°F.

Preheat the broiler or griddle pan.

Slice the peaches in half and remove the pits, trying to keep the cut as clean as possible. Carefully place the peach halves, cut sides down, and grill until each peach half has become slightly charred.

Thinly slice the vanilla bean lengthwise, remove seeds, and put into a mortar with the sugar. Pound with the pestle until broken up and combined.

Place the peach halves cut sides up in a shallow ovenproof baking dish. Scatter the vanilla sugar over the peaches and pour in some of the Amaretto. Place in the preheated oven and bake for 10 minutes or until the peaches are soft.

Pour over the remaining Amaretto and serve hot or cold with (highly optional) crème fraîche.

Serves 6

8 ripe peaches

1 vanilla bean

2 tablespoons sugar (less if you can!)

1/2 cup Amaretto

crème fraîche (optional)

[**Believe me,
if I can do it,
you can do it.**
Ed Victor]

CHAPTER TEN

Happily Ever After:

Making The Obvious Diet Permanent

If the principles of The Obvious Diet are so very obvious, then why write a book about it? Because, as we all know, the obvious frequently needs stating! There is a reason why human beings have traditionally learned things by rote, through repetition followed by more repetition and then exams requiring revision (yet more repetition): it's the way we make things stick. And that's the way I hope you can stick to your very own Obvious Diet. Reconfiguring your appetite is not an impossible task — it's a matter of replacing bad habits with good habits, and the good news is that once you get going, achieving your goals is actually far easier than you might have feared. Though "Obvious" may not be synonymous with "easy" — for me my weight loss, and the slaying of my personal food demons, has been quite an achievement – it is, without doubt, within the possibilities of us all.

Although the good habits of The Obvious Diet will surprisingly quickly replace the bad habits built up over a lifetime, as with cigarettes, you may occasionally long for a smoke. But – and this is the clincher – once you have made your personal investment in your Obvious Diet, you know incontrovertibly how much better off you are by staying the course; what is the appeal of a moment of fleeting gratification compared to the progress you have made? Why lay yourself open to the torment and self-doubt you are so successfully putting behind you?

What underpins every person's individual Obvious Diet – and by this, I mean a balanced and healthy long-term attitude and approach to food in your life – is that you retrain your past habits. What emerges is the reformed character you had always secretly hoped lurked within, but feared would never be able to emerge. Bad food behavior – whether it's binge eating, comfort eating, eating the wrong kinds of foods, or just plain overeating – is not a life sentence, it's something that, with a reasonable amount of work, and with the support of those around you too, you can overcome.

Many people have achieved this before this book was even thought of. I hope that the difference, now, is that there exists a resource that says, in black and white, that your own diet, made and designed and policed by you, is the very best chance you have to find a happy medium between your pre–Obvious Diet body shape and your "ideal" body shape. Believe me, if I can do it, you can do it.

Bad food behavior is not a life sentence, it's something that, with a reasonable amount of work, you can overcome.

Human beings are astonishing. We are capable of the most extraordinary feats. I'm not talking about going to the moon or splitting the atom, but about escaping from deeply ingrained, sometimes lifelong, patterns of behavior. Saying that all it takes is willpower may be simplistic – it is simplistic, but the willpower is fundamental.

The Obvious Diet is yours to draw up as you see fit, yours to follow, and yours to police. One vital factor to success I have mentioned in passing, exercise, is very important to the mix. Exercise and diet go hand in hand. To do one without the other makes no sense. Exercise not only makes you fitter, it burns off excess fat you have built up, reduces stress, provides a sense of achievement as you can do more, more easily, and gives you a clear measure of how far you have come since the bad old days when you were in thrall to your food cravings. Exercise must fit in with your life schedule and be something you enjoy or learn to enjoy, and something you can feasibly do. But it is important that you ease into it. By that, I don't mean going to the gym once every two weeks, or walking to the shops once or twice instead of taking the car: I mean start slowly, with a program that fits in with your capabilities and what you like, ideally after seeking advice from a trainer at your local gym, or else from your GP. Sudden, heavy exercise after a long period of inactivity is almost guar- anteed to result in injury, and what do we tend to do if we are immobi- lized for a while and feeling sorry for ourselves? Bingeing and comfort eating, the very behavior that blows any diet, however strong the good intentions, right out of the water.

Exercise and diet go hand in hand. But it is important that you ease into it.

After you have followed your Obvious Diet for a couple of months, and it has become a familiar feature of your day, it may be illuminating to keep a food diary again for a few days, just to compare how (and what) you are eating now with then. Apart from your Treat Meal – your own personal food cravings safety valve – you should find that what has gone are all the unhealthy, thoughtless but comforting things you used to eat (the things you ate and finished without hardly noticing, only to find moments later that you were headed for the fridge or the pantry to get yet more of the same junk "comfort food").

And then what? What happens three months, six months, a year down the line? If your Obvious Diet works for you anything like it has for me, you might experience a moment similar to me after I passed the nine-month mark. The following exchange took place at my doctor's office during my annual September checkup:

"Get on the scales," said my doctor, Scottish GP Angus Blair.

"No, I don't want to weigh myself," I replied, explaining that I had banished scales as part of my Obvious Diet.

"On the scales, Ed," repeated Dr. Blair in his sternest voice. And you don't disagree with Angus Blair, a fifth-generation physician!

The scales told an interesting tale. What we discovered was that, in September 2001, I weighed 173 pounds, approximately what I had weighed when I was an undergraduate at Dartmouth, at my physical peak, aged 20. Dr. Blair consulted his records for September 2000, the date of my previous birthday checkup; I had weighed 213 pounds, which meant that I had lost a colossal 40 pounds since I embarked on The Obvious Diet in early January. But then I remembered that after my grief-stricken autumn of 2000 I had indulged in a wild bout of comfort eating, and put on a lot of weight … leading to the Epiphany of the Unbuttonable Trousers on New Year's Eve 2001, the moment that I realized the obvious, that things simply had to change. So exactly how much had I weighed, I wondered, when I first began the Obvious Diet? 220 pounds? 225 pounds? Who knew? And, frankly, who cared? All water under the bridge, or more accurately, weight off my frame.

All I knew for sure was that I had lost at least 40 pounds – perhaps even 50 pounds – during the first eight months of following my personal Obvious Diet. This weight loss – and the new sense of my body that

Even The Obvious Diet can benefit from moderation.

accompanied it – went far beyond my wildest dreams and hopes. There in my doctor's office, in my underclothes, the full extent of my weight loss exposed, I have to confess that the thought of what I had achieved filled me with pride.

But my private moment of glory was punctured by a stern admonition from Dr. Blair: "Ed," he said, "absolutely no more weight loss. Keep to this weight, but, please, NO MORE!"

This was not the first such warning I had received. My wife, of all people, had started to complain that I was getting "too thin." She was joined in this complaint by many of our friends and clients, including Nigella Lawson, Ruth Rogers, and Candice Bergen. "You've lost too much weight," they would intone, "we want our 'Big Ed' back!" Even more vociferous was my friend Maurice (now Lord) Saatchi: "Stop! You look emaciated! You have an eating disorder!" he would warn me every time we met. To cap it off, one of the bellmen at the Regency Hotel, where I always stay in New York, put a kindly hand on my arm one day and asked in genuine concern: "Mr. Victor, are you alright?" as if I had contracted some dread illness.

As with anything, you can have too much of a good thing.

What was going on here? Were they all wrong, simply jealous of what I had finally achieved, or did they have a point? Were they indulging that all-too-human trait of fighting against change, or had I really got to the point where I had reached my goal and needed to rethink the details of my Obvious Diet?

The time had come to acknowledge that as with anything, you can have too much of a good thing. Even The Obvious Diet can benefit from moderation. Or, more accurately, modulation. I had reached my desired weight, the general target zone, thanks to the eating patterns I had established through the whole process of setting up and following my Obvious Diet. Clearly I now had a different task at hand: to stop losing weight without putting it back on. To maintain myself at the ideal shape and weight I felt I had reached, I needed to fine-tune the overall framework.

And when you arrive at this juncture, as I fervently hope you do, you might be interested in one or two pointers on how to fine-tune your Obvious Diet and how to cope, sartorially and in other ways, with your new weight and body shape.

Maintaining Your Weight

Eating in order not to gain weight is different from eating in order to lose weight. That much is, as always, a statement of the plainly obvious! Although I have strongly advocated the banishment of scales from the dieting process, the cold hard truth of the scales can have its benefits – in helping you to stay within the range of your ideal weight. And so, contrary to my advice for the initial stages of The Obvious Diet, there is a strong case for monitoring your weight on a weekly basis (not more than that, or it can become unnecessarily obsessive!). You don't need scales during the weight loss phase of your Obvious Diet because, as I have said, watching calibrations slowly count down may actually discourage and inhibit your resolve. You will know without mechanical aids when you have attained the weight and the shape that is ideal for you – the reactions of those around you are as accurate as any set of scales – just as you knew all along exactly how to succeed! But once you reach the Promised Land, you will want to stay there, and not venture any further.

Here are my suggestions for modifying your eating plan when you think you've lost enough weight – note, these are only suggestions: just as you were the best-placed person for working out how to revolutionize your diet in the first place, with the additional experience of conquering your excess weight, you're unbeatable when it comes to tweaking your own personal winning formula!

The Obvious Diet is, above all, a commonsense diet. Keeping to your ideal weight requires only the same common sense that brought you to that weight. Use it! You should choose a regular day of the week on which to weigh yourself ritually; I prefer Monday morning, not just because it is the start of a new week, but because I have usually had my Cleansing Day the day before, so the needle is as low as it's going to go. If you are within a couple of pounds of your desired weight, then just continue to eat as you have been eating. But if there is any significant change (not a pound or two, I mean five pounds or more in either direction) then adjust your eating accordingly for the week.

You might, by the way, at this point enjoy another trawl through your cookbook collection to allow in some of the recipes you rejected when you were adhering to your strict weight loss diet. I don't mean you should go crazy, but, for example, you don't necessarily need to avoid recipes that use a little butter or a little flour. A modicum of a previously banished foodstuff is not going to undo your weight loss ... you've proven yourself to be made of sterner stuff!

At this stage, it's a matter of relaxing from (not abandoning) the rules and stratagems you have devised for your Obvious Diet. Remember, the devil never sleeps, so you must not completely ignore the rules you made when you started: just bend them a little. For example, although you should continue religiously your weekly Cleansing Day ritual, it doesn't have to be as stringent as before. In what ways? Use some vinaigrette (or whatever sauce you like best) on your vegetables. Have a little yogurt, if that is what you like, with your fruit. But don't, please, allow alcohol into your Cleansing Day: it is so good for the body to take at least one day off! You can also allow yourself generally to eat more: if your new dietary habits have limited you to a certain quantity of food, and there's an occasion when you'd really love the indulgence of taking a small second helping of a particularly tasty item, go for it – if you've got this far with your Obvious Diet, a little digression is not going to do you any harm. However, as you will be well aware, The Obvious Diet will, over time, blunt your

I try to focus on my goals every day, because, as I have said, the devil never sleeps!

greed, so that you won't want as much food as you did previously. So let yourself go a little if the moment is right. If you feel like it, have an occasional three-course (instead of the ritual two of The Obvious Diet) meal. Don't allow yourself more than one out-and-out Treat Meal per week, but do allow yourself an occasional nibble of foods you once considered banned. You can risk a bite of a former comfort food without it threatening the whole edifice of your new way of eating. In my own case, for example, I now taste a bit of cheese occasionally, rather than wait for the weekly Treat Meal. You must not relinquish your grip on the central tenets of your diet – what you eat for breakfast, how often and when you eat the things that are your own personal weaknesses (bread or pasta due to my wheat intolerance, for you it could be sweets or fatty meats or cream or fried foods . . .), how much alcohol you consume and when you consume it – but just allow a gentle bending of the previously inviolable rules. By getting this far you have earned the right to trust yourself.

Clothes Maketh

When you lose a lot of weight, it is oh so obvious to your friends. You become an object of great interest, especially at social mealtimes. In the early stages of your Obvious Diet, you are more likely to receive compliments than brickbats, though occasionally some well-meaning friend or family member will say something that seems maliciously designed to undermine your resolve (remember "Go on, one little ＊＊＊＊ won't kill you"?). Once you have achieved your ideal weight a subtle change takes place. At a certain point the initial paeans of praise turn to a chorus of censure. I simply cannot remember the number of times that people have come up to me in a restaurant, seen a blob of sauce on my plate, and in a j'accuse tone said: "You eat THAT?" Equally, they express astonishment when I sip a glass of wine with dinner, as I occasionally do. We all love attention, but after a while this kind of scrutiny can become exhausting. Perhaps it is jealousy that you have stuck to your guns so rigorously, when they may not have been able to break out from the old cyclical patterns of dieting and plumping up again.

It took me a while to realize why, when I felt so svelte and healthy, I began to hear this litany of complaint and concern. Finally, the penny dropped. It was not the amount of weight I had lost – as I write, I still weigh around 175 pounds – but the simple fact that I had not done what I needed to do: go out and buy new clothes! When you shed the kind of weight I did, getting on for a quarter of my old body weight, your body shape changes so much that all your clothes – suits, jacket, trousers, shirts, sweaters, etc. – hang

Reinvent a new you. Change your wardrobe.

off you in such a way as to make you look "emaciated" or even "ill." And wearing clothes that swim on your new shape will encourage your friends to disapprove (or even pity!) you more and more.

Please learn a lesson from me and don't wait too long to change your wardrobe. And I mean change it radically. I made the mistake of wearing the same old clothes, even though they were swimming on me. All this does is make you seem much too thin, even haggard, when exactly the opposite is true, namely that you have achieved your ideal weight and are in fact feeling as fit and well as you have ever felt!

As soon as you get within range of your ideal weight – ideal not just for how you want to look, but for your height and age, as listed in those doctors' tables – another lesson I can pass on is that you are better off buying new clothes than altering old ones. If you have taken off ten or fifteen pounds, then, fine, your clothes can be taken in by the tailor around the corner. But after losing twenty or more pounds, it becomes a case of expensively remaking clothes rather than merely altering them, and that kind of tailoring doesn't come cheap. Therefore, it might make sense not to alter anything other than your best, most expensive clothing and buy the rest afresh.

Take advantage of this golden opportunity, reinvent a new you on the outside to match the new person you feel you are on the inside. In my case, I now buy 36" waist trousers, instead of the 40" waist I needed before The Obvious Diet. My suit size has gone from 46 long to 44 or even 42 long. And my neck has shrunk from 17" to 16" and then 15½". For men, having the right size shirt is very important; a collar that hangs off your neck makes you look ill. Shirts are not by any means the most expensive item in your wardrobe, so go on a shirt-buying spree as soon as you can after your weight has leveled off – it's fun to do and will keep you looking healthy and well. Women who may in the past have favored more flowing styles can take the risk of buying more figure-shaped items, or expand the range of styles they have by adding skirts or dresses they haven't dared to buy in years.

You don't have to be a rocket scientist to figure out that by throwing out the old and making a major investment in new clothes you also lock yourself into your Obvious Diet plan for the future. The consequences, both financial and emotional, of allowing your old weight to creep back on, are reinforced! The day you really burn your bridges with the past is the day that you donate your old wardrobe to charity.

So, enjoy the fruits (and vegetables and reasoned eating patterns) of all your labors. And while you don't need to adhere as slavishly as you did to the letter of rules you evolved, you do need to keep them going in spirit. Which is precisely what you've been retraining yourself for all along! I still largely stick to fruit, and only fruit, for breakfast, grilled chicken or fish with vegetables or salads for lunch and dinner.

I allow myself modest amounts of sauce – always noticed by my dining companions with mock horror! – and don't inhibit myself when I crave a little more food. But the maintenance phase is easier and more pleasurable than I had ever imagined, because, by now, as I hope you have had a chance to experience for yourself, sticking to the basic principles of The Obvious Diet is not just "second nature," it's your true nature.

Recipe Index

Dressing and Sauces

Acknowledgments

When I first crossed the mysterious border from being a publisher to being an agent in 1974, people said I was a "poacher turned game-keeper." Now that I have momentarily crossed the border from representing authors to actually being one myself, I suppose I could be said to be a "gamekeeper turned game"! My newest perspective on the book trade has made me more aware than ever of just how many people are involved in the supposedly individual act of creating a book. My thanks are due, therefore, to far more people than space would allow me to mention on this page. But here goes:

I never thought I would be thanking one of my chief rivals for helping me, but Jonathan Lloyd has been a model advocate for me and my book, as well as an astute deal-maker and advisor.

My British publishers at Vermilion could not have been more encouraging while I was writing this book or more efficient after it was handed in. Everyone connected with the publishing process there, including but not limited to Gail Rebuck, Amelia Thorpe, Denise Bates, Sarah Bennie, and Helen Marriage, has earned my gratitude and my admiration – which I must confess is not always the case between the authors I represent and their publishers! At the risk of being invidious, however, I must single out Denise Bates, a great hands-on editor who was unfailingly there for me at every point in this nerve-wracking process!

Jeannette and Dick Seaver of Arcade have been enthusiasts about this book ever since they first heard of it. The fact that such old, dear friends are publishing my first book in the U.S. is an immense joy to me ... and, by becoming one of their authors, I have now found out first-hand that their skills match their passion for publishing! I have also been wisely counseled about the pleasures and perils of publishing my book in the U.S. by Sandi Mendelson and Judy Hilsinger, the best book publicists in the business, and by Michael Viner and Deborah Raffin, my long-standing pals and collaborators, now happily my audio publishers.

My friends have rallied around me most magnificently, as I lost pounds and simultaneously accumulated pages for my book. I am tremendously grateful to all my pals who contributed their diet secrets and recipes: Sir Ranulph Fiennes, Ken Follett, Tina Brown, Rose Gray, Marie Helvin, Erica Jong, Larry King, Andrew Lloyd Webber, Nan Kempner, David and Patsy Puttnam, Anne Robinson, Ruth Rogers, Sidney Sheldon, Koo Stark, Art Cooper, Mel Brooks, and Anne Bancroft. Very special thanks are due here to my friends and clients Ruth Rogers and Rose Gray, whose magnificent River Cafe Cookbooks provide the bedrock of the recipe section in *The Obvious Diet.*

My gratitude to Nigella Lawson for writing the foreword, at a par-ticularly busy and stressful period of her life, knows no bounds. How she has managed to do this so eloquently and elegantly – in addition to everything else she does! – will always remain a mystery to me.

An equally deep mystery is how Larry King does all he does ... and still can find the time to write the introduction to this book. He epitomizes the phrase, "if you want something done, ask a busy person." And there is no one busier than Larry!

Huge thanks also to Dr. Mosaraf Ali, not only for the extremely practical advice I have quoted extensively in the book, but also for inspiring me to lead a healthier – and therefore happier – existence.

I was helped and supported throughout by my colleagues at Ed Victor Ltd, notably Linda Van, Lizzy Kremer, Maggie Phillips, Sophie Hicks, Hitesh Shah, and Gráinne Fox.

My family – my wife, Carol, my sons, Adam, Ivan, and Ryan, and my daughters-in-law, Patrizia and Sophie – have cheered me on enthusiastically from the sidelines, both in what I was trying to achieve for myself with my diet and in the intense process of getting it all down on paper.

Lastly, but probably most significantly, I literally could not have produced this book without the brilliant editorial collaboration of my son Adam Victor. His eagle eyes scrutinized every word in every paragraph on every page of this book, and he cut me absolutely no slack just because I'm his dad! A large part of my enjoyment and sense of satisfaction in writing this book came from working and sharing with him. May we collaborate on another book soon!

The author and publishers would like to extend their thanks for permission to quote from the following titles:

Ali, Dr. Mosaraf. *The Integrated Health Bible*, Vermilion, 2001.

Beard, James. *American Cookery*, Little, Brown & Company, 1980.

Child, Julia, Louiselle Bertholle, and Simone Beck, *Mastering the Art of French Cooking*, Vols. 1–2, Knopf, 2001.

Cunningham, Marion, Lauren Jarrett (Illustrator), and Fannie Merrit Farmer. *Fannie Farmer Cookbook*, Knopf, 1996.

Fiennes, Sir Ranulph. *Fit for Life*, Little, Brown & Company, 1998.

Gray, Ruth, and Ruth Rogers. *The Cafe Cookbook*, Broadway, 1998.

———. *River Cafe Cookbook Green*, Ebury, 2000.

———. *The Rogers Gray Italian Country Cookbook*, Random House, 1996.

Hopkinson, Simon. *Roast Chicken and Other Stories*, Ebury, 1999.

Kerkhofs, Eddie. *Le Dome at Home: Great Menus for Entertaining from the Chef/Proprietor of Le Dome Restaurant*, Doubleday, 1996.

Lawson, Nigella. *Nigella Bites*, Chatto and Windus, 2001.

Lawson, Nigella. *How to Eat*, John Wiley & Co., 2000.

Meyer, Danny and Michael Romano. *The Union Square Café Cookbook*, HarperCollins Publishers, 1994.

Stewart, Martha. *The Martha Stewart Cookbook: Collected Recipes for Every Day*, Random House, 1995.

The Ladies Village Improvement Society of East Hampton, Inc. *The East Hampton Cookbook*.

Index